HEALING
DEPRESSION
NATURALLY

HEALING
DEPRESSION
NATURALLY

Lewis Harrison

<small>FOREWORD BY JACK CANFIELD</small>

TWIN STREAMS
Kensington Publishing Corp.
http://www.kensingtonbooks.com

This book presents information based upon the research and personal experiences of the author. It is not intended to be a substitute for a professional consultation with a physician or other healthcare provider. Neither the publisher nor the author can be held responsible for any adverse effects or consequences resulting from the use of any of the information in this book. They also cannot be held responsible for any errors or omissions in the book. If you have a condition that requires medical advice, the publisher and author urge you to consult a competent healthcare professional.

Trademarked and registered names are used in an editorial fashion only in this book. Rather than put a trademark or registration symbol after every occurrence of such a name, we have printed the names with initial caps. These names are used in this book for the benefit of the trademark or registration owner and with no intention of infringement of the trademark or registration.

TWIN STREAMS BOOKS are published by

Kensington Publishing Corp.
850 Third Avenue
New York, NY 10022

All Kensington titles, imprints, and distributed lines are available at special quantity discounts for bulk purchases for sales promotion, premiums, fund-raising, educational or institutional use.

Special book excerpts or customized printings can also be created to fit specific needs. For details, write or phone the office of the Kensington Special Sales Manager: Kensington Publishing Corp., 850 Third Avenue, New York, NY 10022. Attn. Special Sales Department. Phone: 1-800-221-2647.

Twin Streams and the TS logo Reg. U.S. Pat. & TM Off.

ISBN 0-7582-0538-4

First Trade Printing: September 2004
10 9 8 7 6 5 4 3 2 1

Printed in the United States of America

To Spaulding Gray whose
art brought light to all of us
and
To my wife, Lilia, who can bring virtually
anyone out of a depression
just by her presence of being.

CONTENTS

FOREWORD

Depression is not a selective disease. This awful disease can affect an individual of any race, religion, nation, economic class, or political persuasion. Composer Cole Porter fell into a deep depression in the late 1940s that plagued him to his death in 1964. Winston Churchill suffered through most of his life in a struggle with depression that he came to call "the black dog." Buzz Aldrin, the second man to walk on the moon, began suffering from a type of depression he called "the melancholy of things done." The great writer and storyteller Mark Twain suffered from a period of great depression toward the end of his life. Abraham Lincoln, considered by many to be the greatest of all American presidents, suffered throughout his life from what was then called melancholy. Poet Emily Dickinson wrote a poem about an emotional breakdown she experienced, saying, "I felt a funeral in my brain."

Depression often seems to have a life of its own. Like some creature from one of those *Alien* movies, it grows inside you and begins to consume you. Friends and family want to help and offer support, but what they say just doesn't get in. When you are depressed, you feel completely isolated. Depressed individuals sincerely want help and yet they often seem paralyzed in acting on that desire. People with the best of intentions will tell you to "get on with your life," "snap out of it," "think positive," and "exercise!" It isn't as easy as that. Depression, and the treatment of its symptoms, is both basic and highly complex at the same time.

Depression has become one of the major health problems in recent years. With the advent of technology, such as the Internet, e-mail, faxes, and wireless devices, we are being forced to work harder than ever bebre, to be on call longer, while at the same time, to take less vacation and personal time. Catastrophic world events have only exacerbated this, pawning a record number of new cases of depression. In 2001, the National Book Award Winner in the category of Nonfiction—and a major bestseller—was a book about depression.

Unfortunately, it is predicted only to get worse. In 2002, almost 20 million Americans were diagnosed with some form of clinical depression. The World Health Organization predicts that by the year 2020, five of the ten leading medical problems worldwide will be stress related.

Most mental health professionals over the years have seen depression purely as a state of mind. In the last four decades, research has indicated that there are many forces at work that ultimately lead to depression.

Simultaneously, the use of nutritional products and herbal preparations by the general public is one of the fastest-growing segments in consumer spending and in health care. In 1993, Dr. David Eisenberg, a professor at Harvard University, published the first of two important studies showing that one in three Americans had used some form of alternative medicine.

Recent medical studies have indicated that various noninvasive approaches have the ability to bring short-term and, in many cases, permanent relief from this debilitating emotional disorder. Research in recent years has also shown that depression is seldom isolated. It is generally experienced with other symptoms, which might include headache, subclinical nutritional deficiencies, digestive problems, and insomnia. These are all conditions that can be positively influenced by nutrition, herbs, amino acid supplementation, hands-on healing, specialized counseling and coaching systems, and other approaches either alone or, when necessary, in combination with medication.

Lewis Harrison's book *Healing Depression Naturally* presents a well-organized, step-by-step program that integrates nutrition, homeopathy, amino acid therapy, herbal-based healing techniques (including flower remedies and aromatherapy), hands-on healing, healing through movement, color and music therapy, intestinal detoxification, glandular balancing, behavior modification, and ancient approaches that have been used in China and India for thousands of years. Lewis has included personal testimonies from those who have escaped from the dark cloud of depression or have learned to live with it while experiencing life fully in spite of the constant presence.

This is not meant to be a scholarly work. Lewis has avoided using the technical language used in many scientific and medical journals. This book is for both the physician and the patient. In it you will learn to cleanse the blood and subtly influence brain chemistry by balancing glandular function. By addressing the nervous system, the program ensures proper healing of emotional issues that might lead to depression, with a coordination of the elimination and rebuilding functions. The program is designed to help you move beyond a depressed state while relaxing and regenerating nerve and muscle tissue, improving cellular absorption of oxygen and other nutrients, strengthening intestinal muscles, improving peristalsis, and increasing bowel evacuation to bring about the gradual cleansing of the intestinal tract. Following this program may have an immediate impact on your mental and physical health, and lead you to the threshold of a greatly improved quality of life.

Long-term chronic depression, more often than not, is managed rather than cured. Even so, a key step in climbing out of the darkness of depression is in understanding that this depression is not who you are but rather an illness that you are experiencing. It has symptoms, causes, and solutions. Thanks to both huge advances in the study of nutrition, herbology, and brain chemistry, which Harrison covers so thoroughly and clearly, and the growing popularity of integrative, holistic approaches, which take into account biochemical, emotional, cultural, structural, and spiritual factors, hope exists for more effective therapy with more successful outcomes than have ever resulted before. The emergence of new information as well as the availability of health professionals with more open attitudes toward new approaches for the treatment of depression together offer a new direction. The real possibility that you can feel better in as little as a few weeks and that you can eliminate or radically reduce future depressive episodes does exist. You can make it your own reality, and Harrison shows you how.

Jack Canfield, coauthor of the
Chicken Soup for the Soul series

PREFACE

Depression. Every day there is another report, study, or viewpoint presented about this subject. With so many different positions on depression even among the experts, it is not difficult to understand why there is so much confusion about the best course of action to take concerning this issue.

For these reasons, when the opportunity arose for me to write *Healing Depression Naturally*, I was very excited. The task of clarifying the misconceptions that people have about natural healing for depression seemed like a worthy endeavor. This book is the result of my desire to convey accurate and helpful information about this important subject.

Mental health is an ever-changing field of study, and an in-depth discussion of nutrition, herbs, glandular function, and brain chemistry could easily become technical. Although there is certainly no shortage of written material on depression, I felt there was a need to write a book that explains the basic causes of and treatments for depression in laymen's terms and to guide you, the reader, in using this information wisely.

As you apply the information presented in *Healing Depression Naturally*, you may find that this entire area of healing falls somewhere between the realms of art and science. By applying the information in this book, you will be able to make clearer and more educated decisions about your personal health and about the health of those who are close to you.

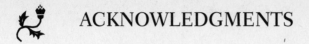

ACKNOWLEDGMENTS

My deepest thanks to Donna Gianell, a faculty member at the Academy of Natural Healing and the former copublisher (with her husband Ken) of *Dance and the Arts* magazine, for her contributions to the section on dance and movement as well as her invaluable editing skill. Thanks to John Beaulieu, Ph.D., for his invaluable assistance on the section describing music, sound, and depression and for his information on tuning forks; Dr. Daniel J. Wiener, for his work on treating depression with Rehearsals for Growth; Sara Vogeler and John Duggan, for their contribution on thyroid testing and progestrone-estrogen imbalances; Debra Burrell, for her contribution on male and female issues and their relationship to depression; to my sister Lily, for her gift of kindness and joy in the most depressing of circumstances; to the faculty and students of the Academy of Natural Healing, for providing the foundation of my work. To Marc Becker at *New Life* magazine, and Paul English at *New York Spirit* magazine, for providing platforms for getting the word out; and to Mary Campbell Gallagher and Jerry Mundis, for their friendship and support at a trying time. To my agent, Noah Lukeman, for his support in creating this project format, and to Kensington's senior editor, Elaine Will Sparber, for her organizational and editing skills. My appreciation to the teachers at Dera Baba Jaimal Singh in Beas, India, for their guidance through the years. Last but not least, to my mother, Dorothy, who at eighty-seven years of age is more unsinkable than can be imagined.

1 WHAT IS DEPRESSION?

Depression is the most commonly experienced emotional disorder and has been with us since the beginning of time. It has been known by many names, including despair and melancholy. One of the reasons why this condition is so widespread is, in no small part, due to the fact that the term *depression* encompasses a wide range of physical and psychological symptoms. In its most extreme forms, suicide is a major risk of depression.

Public perception and medical approaches to depression are determined by complex interactions among the public, the media, politicians, and the medical establishment. Depression appears in many forms and at many levels of severity. In the early stages of the condition, a person may experience a single symptom or a combination of symptoms that have come to be associated with depression. These symptoms may include loss of appetite, loss of interest in hobbies, various sleep disturbances (including insomnia), and loss of sex drive, among others. Having these symptoms does not necessarily mean that a person is in a depressed state. We all experience life events and obstacles that challenge our mental and emotional balance. Healthy grief and depression owing to extreme events may last a few weeks or even longer. Normally, a person will eventually come out of the trauma. But some do not. These individuals seem to sink deeper into a swirl of seemingly ever darker symptoms. When these symptoms last longer than three weeks or a month, and the individual experiences a weight loss of more than 5 percent, and/or is fatigued, has a loss of hope, a sense of despair, and slow and/or distorted thinking, then this individual may be experiencing clinical depression.

There are many different categories of depression. These include chronic depression, bipolar disorder, seasonal affective disorder, postpartum depression, and more recently classified forms of depression such as atypical depression and double depression. Some of these conditions are either biochemical or attitudinal in origin, while others are combinations of the two.

The most common forms are known as situational depression and clinical depression. The difference between the two is defined by the severity and length of time of the depressed state, as well as certain biochemical factors that may have come into play.

To understand how pervasive depression is in the United States and increasingly throughout the world, you need only look at research findings and statistics:

- It is estimated that between 2 and 4 percent of the United States population suffers from some form of clinical depression. The figures are even greater among specialized populations such as the confined elderly, hospital inpatients (especially those in life-challenging situations), patients under primary care, and the chronically ill.
- About twice as many women as men suffer from clinical depression, except for bipolar disorder, which occurs with equal frequency in both genders.
- The largest amount of depression occurs between the ages of twenty-five and forty-four, with an increased rate among those born since 1945.
- Individuals with a family history of depression are more inclined to develop depression.
- Research shows that one in ten people in the United States suffers from depression. However, nearly two-thirds do not get help or treatment because these symptoms are never properly diagnosed.
- "Siblings, parents and children of those with recurrent depression develop mood disorders at eight times the rate of the general population," according to a *Psychology Today* newsletter about depression.[1]

In this chapter, we will review what depression is by examining some of the major forms of the disorder. We will also discuss how depression is diagnosed.

Depression in the Elderly

One of the myths around aging is that depression is a normal aspect of being old. Symptoms such as pessimism, excessive criticism of others, hopelessness concerning the future, and sudden irritability, which are often seen as the "grumpy" personality qualities of the elderly, are all symptoms of clinical depression.

Depression often goes undetected in the elderly because patients do not report their symptoms, and those who recognize the problem may attempt to self-treat. Many older adults resist diagnosis and treatment due to the stigma connected to mental illness in the past, myth-based fear, lack of information, and misinformation. When doctors recognize these symptoms, they often misinterpret them as some other form of mental illness.

As an older person becomes frail, they will sometimes exhibit such symptoms as loss of appetite, fatigue, and a lack of interest in things that were formerly sources of great pleasure. All of these are symptoms of depression.

In 1995, Dr. Barry Liebowitz, chief of the Mental Disorders Among the Aging Research Branch at the National Institute of Mental Health. estimated that of the over 32 million Americans aged sixty-five and older, as many as 6 million suffered from some form of clinical depression, and of these, at least 75 percent went undiagnosed and untreated. According to Dr. Liebowitz, the prognosis for elderly patients whose depression is diagnosed and treated is good. "We know that treatment works in 80% of cases where patients receive appropriate treatment."[2]

Mitral Valve Prolapse

Mitral valve prolapse, often found in thin, young women, involves a leaky heart valve, often resulting from hardened tissue, possibly tiny calcium deposits, in the valves. Many believe it is nutritionally caused by mineral imbalances, particularly of magnesium. Because it affects circulation and flow of oxygen in the brain, depression often arises when this condition is present.

Situational Depression

Researchers know that certain experiences in a person's life such as childhood sexual abuse, being bullied at school, and other similar situations are more likely to result in depressive episodes than others. These factors can also include typical grief reactions to incapacitating clinical depression.

A stable, highly functional individual with what would be considered a normal personality may experience a crisis or other triggering event that may result in depression. This situational type of depression may be triggered by such common occurrences as separation or divorce, work failure, physical illness, or confusion in one's sexual identity. Sometimes an individual can become depressed after suffering a physical injury if he or she has not responded as well as the person expected to traditional therapeutic approaches such as speech, occupational, or physical therapy. Their sense of hopelessness and helplessness can affect sleeping and eating patterns and create a dark cloud over the person's life.

Depression can also be triggered by a stressful personal event such as a change of circumstances or the loss of a loved one. Short-term depression is a normal means of coping with such situations. However, chronic forms of depression may be caused by innumerable factors. The most common causes include subclinical nutritional deficiencies, brain chemical imbalances, an underlying disease (such as hepatitis C), food allergy (particularly gluten intolerance), Wilson's disease, immune problems, blood sugar metabolism disorders, adverse reaction to medications, as well as hormonal imbalance (particularly hypothyroidism and pancreatic insufficiency), low cholesterol, sensitivity to environmental chemicals, and other environmental factors including high positive ion levels. Each of these conditions requires professional care.

Depression is not a sign of personal failure at the game of life. In fact, many highly successful people, including the actor Rod Steiger, writer William Styron, journalist Mike Wallace, and writer-newspaper columnist Art Buchwald, have all publicly revealed that they suffer from depression.

My good friend Jerrold Mundis is a writer who has published forty novels and books of nonfiction, including selections by the Book-of-the-Month Club, Literary Guild, and One Spirit Book Club. He also coaches writers from beginners to best-selling authors, and breaks writer's block—forever—for people in a single afternoon consultation. Just as significantly, for our purposes, Jerry has had to cope with depression through his entire adult life. I asked him to tell me what depression is like for him. He said:

> It sucks joy and color out of your life. Everything becomes flat, gray, dead. Nothing means anything. You have no energy, no will. You can't

move. You can't answer the phone. Simply walking across a room can seem like a monumental, even impossible, task. I once went three days just sitting on the couch, not turning on the lights, not doing anything.

At its best, when the depression is low level, you're stale and lethargic. You can't get interested in anything. Everything just seems too difficult. You're uncommunicative, listless. You *can't* respond, *can't* take action on your own behalf. That's what people around you don't understand. They say, "Come out to a movie with me," or "Why don't you go for a good walk in the sunlight." Yes, those things might well help some, but you just can't bring yourself to do them—that's part of the nature of depression.

In a serious depression, everything seems utterly hopeless. You feel only pain and despair: overwhelming, total annihilation. You can't remember that anything ever felt any different. You can't conceive that it ever will feel any different. It is agony. It is very nearly unbearable, and for some, crosses over the line. Most depressives who kill themselves don't really want to die—they just want the pain to stop, *need* the pain to stop, can't stand it anymore. And suicide is the only answer they can find. I've come very close to it two, maybe three, different times myself because of depression.[3]

These are chilling words, especially from someone for whom you care. But I also know Jerry as a man who functions well in life and even helps others to do that, too. I asked him how he managed to deal with his depression, how he continues to manage. He said:

I have a mix of techniques and strategies, which I developed mostly by trial and error. The first thing that truly helped me was cognitive psychology. I am convinced that the only forms of psychotherapy that can even *touch* depression are cognitive psychology as developed by Dr. Aaron Beck and, to a somewhat lesser degree, rational-emotive therapy as developed by Dr. Albert Ellis.

There came a time, though, when that failed, too. Years earlier, I had been in a depression study at Columbia-Presbyterian Hospital in New York. They still had all my medical workups. I went back there, consulted with one of their psychopharmacologists, and finally consented to go on medication, though I was leery of it. I was afraid of becoming dulled or affectless, which would be disastrous for a writer (on the other hand, my depressions were already that). I went on Prozac. What the Prozac did was act as a kind of safety net, which kept me from plunging down completely into darkness and despair when I was in a decline. But it was never fully reliable. We had to keep tinkering with the dose and experimenting with other antidepressants, none of which worked for me.

After several years, grateful for the Prozac, but never truly comfortable or even reliably steadied with it, and after a bit of research, I decided to go off Prozac and try the nutritional supplement SAM-e [S-adenosyl-methionine], which is used as a prescription antidepressant in some European countries, but which can be purchased over the counter here. It was very successful. I have found SAM-e much more helpful and effective, for me, than Prozac. I don't have to tinker with the dose much, my mood is more stable than it was with Prozac, and there are virtually no side effects.

I also use light. I have a strong element of SAD [seasonal affective disorder] in my depression. It's not the totality by any means, but it does play a strong role. Unaddressed, the diminishing light of winter will have me on the floor, with beginning suicidal ideation, by winter solstice, no matter what other measures I'm taking. I use light in two guises: first, every bulb in my home is a full-spectrum bulb (and that's year round). If I am in dim light or even normal incandescent light in winter, I can actually feel my mood begin to slip. Second, I use a light box—commercially manufactured to treat SAD—through which I expose my face (it's light entering the eyes that is significant) to high-intensity light for a given period each day during the winter months. I've used a light box for some eight years now, and it's made a significant, positive difference.

So there you have it. I hope my own experience will be helpful to others. Depression is a hellish condition and I wish relief from it for everyone who has ever suffered from it.[4]

Whew! Thank you, Jerry.

Most of us believe that it is the external circumstances and events of our lives that influence mood. The truth is, mood is also influenced by attitude. This factor of "attitude" is more than just a psychological state. Attitude is, to a large degree, a response to complex biochemical processes that give one reaction or another greater importance. Luckily, as complex as all of these interacting variables are, science has identified many of the biological conditions that most greatly influence mood changes.

Depression often appears as a response to illness. It is natural for physicians and other healthcare workers to view depression or stress in patients as a normal and healthy response to life-challenging events like a stroke, a heart attack, or cancer. However, there is a thin line that separates a normal sense of anxiety, stress, and a feeling of "the blues" from a serious clinical depression. Sometimes, in fact, the former may mask the latter. When this is the case, depression may interfere with a patient's recovery.

According to Dr. Rex W. Cowdry, acting director of the National Institute of Mental Health, "When the depressed mood is fixed and pervasive, and severely interferes with normal function, it's something that should be recognized and evaluated as possibly a separate clinical entity."[5]

Post-traumatic stress disorder (PTSD) is a specific type of situational depression that occurs in and after an intensely stressful event such as an experience in the military or police services, terrorism, a major accident, or schoolyard bullying.

To help determine if your depression is situational, see "Is Your Depression Situational or Biochemical?" below.

Is Your Depression Situational or Biochemical?

Though they may actually blend together, there are distinctive aspects of a biochemically based depression that distinguish it from situational depression (depression that stems from emotional trauma and from negative life events). There is a good chance that a depression is biochemical in origin if any of the following factors describes this depression:

- You cannot remember or identify any specific time, date, or event that marked the onset of your depression.
- You awaken very early in the morning and are unable to go back to sleep.
- You experience extreme mood swings between depression and elation over a period of a few months. (This suggests bipolar disorder.)
- You have been depressed for a month or longer even though you have made many positive changes in your life.
- Heavy drinking and substance abuse make your depression worse.
- Good news or positive events in your life seem to have no effect on you.
- Analysis, talk therapy or other psychotherapy approaches have little or no effect. This is even more so if psychological probing—questions like, "How do you feel about your mother?"—or if talking about unresolved childhood issues leaves you overwhelmed and confused.

Postpartum Depression

When an ordinary, healthy person experiences stress, the hypothalamus secretes corticotrophin-releasing hormone (CRH). CRH then triggers the release of certain hormones, which increase the cortisol levels in the blood.

This is important because stress affects blood pressure and blood sugar, and the hormone cortisol helps maintain normal levels of both. Not only are cortisol levels directly related to the amount of CRH released from the hypothalamus, but the thyroid hormone, which is involved in the regulation of mood, is influenced by cortisol levels as well. During the last trimester of pregnancy, CRH is released by the placenta into the mother's bloodstream, increasing blood CRH levels to three times what would be considered normal.

After birth and removal of the placenta, the mother's CRH commonly drops to levels seen in people showing clinical signs of depression. It is generally believed that the excess CRH produced by the placenta suppresses the production of CRH by the mother's hypothalamus. After childbirth, CRH production returns to normal but not quickly enough to maintain emotional stability.

During the two or more weeks that it takes for the hypothalamus to return to a normal level of CRH, the new mother may experience "the blues"—postpartum depression (PPD).

Women who suffer from PPD may become paralyzed with fear and concern for the safety of their baby. If there is a PPD concern, seek professional support and diagnosis to distinguish this from other conditions such as obsessive-compulsive disorder. Though not all women experience this problem, 12 to 16 percent do, and, according to some experts, extreme forms can include a "break" with reality—a loss of the ability to discern what is real from what is not. Researchers believe that the mothers who avoid this type of depression recover the ability to regulate CRH more quickly than the ones who experience "baby blues."

Hormones and Depression

Hormones are substances produced by several glands and organs in your body such as the thyroid, testes, ovaries, pancreas, liver, and pituitary. Secreted directly from where they are produced into the bloodstream, each hormone has a specific function, which it accomplishes by interacting with its receptors. Each hormone plays a key role in the maintenance of brain health. Some hormones function as neurotransmitters, sending information to a specific population of brain cells.

Hormones also function as nerve growth factors that guarantee the stimulation, maturation, and connections between brain cells. Hormones differ from enzymes in that the former initiate reactions in the body, whereas the latter usually help to facilitate those reactions. Among the functions of hormones are the regulation of mineral metabolism, reproductive functions, aging, fluid retention, sexual function and libido, and growth and development. Any unbalanced shift in hormonal levels can result in various health problems, including depression. An example of this is premenstrual syndrome (PMS).

The sex hormones estrogen and progesterone are usually in a state of imbalance in PMS. PMS can lead to low blood sugar–based depression, as well as hormonally based depression. These hormone levels can be assessed by way of saliva samples. If an imbalance is found, a combination of dietary intervention, light therapy, hormone-influencing herbs, and hormone augmentation is the most effective form of treatment.

Gender and Depression

It is hard to specifically define the level of depression in certain gender, age, and cultural groups. Depression involves many factors, and different segments of the population have differing ways of relating to and expressing feelings of depression. According to Harvard psychologist William Pollack, Ph.D., young males in the United States, for instance, are culturally influenced early on to suppress feeling or communicating any emotional suffering they might experience.

Most statistics indicate that depression affects women over men two to one. However, it is possible that this statistic is flawed since men are more likely than women to hide their depression.

"Boys are trained in ways that make it likely they get depression later," according to the *Psychology Today* newsletter about depression. "If it doesn't destroy their relationships sooner, it shows up by midlife. Midlife crisis is a euphemism for male-based depression."[6]

Most experts agree that what triggers depression in females is often different from what triggers the condition in males. In addition to this, females and males express depression differently.

When females experience depression, it does not usually happen until adolescence. "Girls who mature early have higher rates of depression than other boys and girls throughout junior and senior high," continues the *Psychology Today* newsletter. No one is sure why this is so, but some researchers believe that a combination of factors including socialization factors, emotional coping habits, generic factors, and neurohormones, such as estrogen, may have an influence.[7]

Recent research reestablishes the belief that there is a difference between men and women not only physically, but emotionally and mentally as well. Men and women use language, react to stress, seek out leisure activities, and even respond to mental health issues differently. As the immensely popular book by Ph.D. John Gray says, "Men Are from Mars, Women Are from Venus."

According to Debra Burrell, C.S.W., a marital therapist practicing in New York City, depression can also relate to people's sense of self-worth. And men and women have different criteria for determining their self-worth. Men value results. They tend to be performance-oriented and value what they accomplish, what can be measured. They use a hierarchical system with the best at the top. "He who has the most toys wins." The need to achieve is connected with the need to feel good about oneself. Men like to solve problems, compete, and win. They tend to be more concerned with world events and their role in it.

The self-esteem of a woman is more often based upon the quality of her relationships. If a woman has satisfying relationships, she may be less stressed than a man if she is not financially successful. Women value sharing, cooperative efforts, and validation—not for what they've done but for who they are. Women are more likely to seek personal validation instead of validation for what they have accomplished. They are more often the homemakers, even if they are employed outside of the home.

A man will take pride in the results of his actions. It's the "bottom line" that counts. When a man makes a lot of money, he tends to feel pretty good about himself. But in an era of financial and economic uncertainty, it is more difficult for a man to solidify his sense of self. If there is no quick-and-easy solution—and if it is something that takes years to build—it is harder for a man to hang on and accept the lack of return on his efforts.

A woman will take pride from the depth and the meaning of her relationships. Even if her team lost, if she felt she made "lifelong friends," then it was a winning situation. Financially, even if a woman fails, if she has someone who loves her, if she is in love and connected to those around her, it is easier for her to regroup and eventually try again.

According to Ms. Burrell, someone who is depressed tends to have a negative and often unrealistic view of him- or herself in the world.

Seasonal Affective Disorder

All life on our planet has adapted to and is nourished by light from the sun and sky, a critical balance of visible color and invisible ultraviolet wavelengths. Over the ages, virtually every living thing developed with the help of nature's full spectrum.

Today, many people suffer from sunlight starvation. As winter approaches and there is less daylight, some people experience a form of depression that disappears during the spring and summer months. It is known as seasonal affective disorder, or SAD. SAD affects four times as many women as men. Sometimes called "the winter blues."

SAD is most common in temperate climates where people spend so much time indoors that they are unable to get their daily requirements for sunlight. People need the full spectrum of light that comes with sunshine. It's vital to life and health. Deprivation of sunlight is not just a winter phenomenon. It can be caused by many factors, including some ordinary behaviors.

One way to avoid sunlight starvation is through full-spectrum indoor lighting. This type of light simulates the full color and beneficial ultraviolet spectrum of sunlight. The full visible and ultraviolet spectrum of natural white light promotes healing benefits as no artificial light can. Look for full-spectrum lightbulbs at your local health-food store, hardware store, or light fixtures store.

The use of full-spectrum lighting indoors has been shown to be very beneficial. Some individuals require full-spectrum light of an intensity that is greater than can be provided by a lightbulb. These individuals use a high-intensity "light box" to get the amount of light they require to be healthy. Perhaps this is due to the fact that light therapy stimulates the production of vitamin D_3, the same type of vitamin D produced by the action of sunlight on the skin. It is important to make note of the fact that vitamin D_3 is required for the proper utilization of magnesium. Magnesium deficiency is a factor in various conditions that cause or contribute to depression. In fact, it is now known that aging is a risk factor for magnesium deficiency. And magnesium deficiency is a major cause of depression.

Although the cause of SAD has not been clinically proven, many treatments seem to have a positive effect on the condition, including amino acids, vitamins, light therapy, negative ions, color therapy, and magnesium supplementation.

Note: Taking 400–600 milligrams of magnesium as magnesium glycinate in the morning and at night may result in a faster recovery from SAD.

Michael Terman, Ph.D., director of the winter depression program at Columbia-Presbyterian Medical Center in New York City states, "Using bright-light therapy to shift the internal circadian clock is the most effective intervention we know about. But proper timing is critical."[8] Dr. Terman has demonstrated that the best time to use bright-light therapy is approximately two and a half to four hours past the midpoint of sleep. By timing the light in this manner, the antidepressant response can be doubled as compared to the effect of using light therapy at any other time of the day.

Caution: Though some people have used melatonin supplements to help with irregular sleep that may be associated with depression, this is contraindicated for those suffering from SAD. For these individuals, melatonin has been found to aggravate their symptoms.

Recreational Drug Use and Depression

Recreational drug use, including marijuana (pot), alcohol, heroin, and cocaine, may cause a susceptible individual to become chronically depressed. Though some of these substances will have greater effects than others, the fact remains that many mental disorders, including depression, are a result of problems with brain chemistry. Recreational drugs create the feelings that they do through the way they influence brain chemistry. About 25 percent of those with major depression have a diagnosable substance abuse problem, and those with substance abuse problems are four and a half times as likely to have mental disorders.[9]

Unlike many other substances that enter the body, drugs and alcohol are able to cross the blood-brain barrier. By crossing this barrier, they can interfere with electrical chemical pathways and central nervous system transmissions by accessing brain cells and damaging their delicate structure. Alcohol is known to rapidly deplete docoshexaenoic acid (DHA), an essential fatty acid required for proper brain functioning. Alcohol also destroys essential precursor amino acids. This may be the reason why alcoholics are so emotionally unbalanced and depressed. Without adequate amino-acid conversion, neurotransmitters can no longer be produced in sufficient amounts; depression and other emotionally based symptoms are the result of this alcoholism-based amino acid deficiency.

Depression as a Personality Disorder

We each possess an individual personality, and it is through this personality that we experience life.

Personality is a key factor in whether or not a person will be depressed. Personality can be defined as an outward character, disposition, and temperament. A person's nature—their identity, individuality, and distinctiveness—is also a key factor in depression.

Each of us has unique traits and patterns of behavior. These traits and patterns enable us to make assumptions of how others will act in different situations. There have been many systems for analyzing and defining personality through the ages. The ancients used astrology, Hippocrates described temperaments, Freud discussed them, and Carl G. Jung, the psychiatric pioneer, described various psychological types. The study of personality is not an exact science. In fact, there are many different systems of viewing personality including the traditional Freudian psychiatric approach, the Jungian approach, Myer-Briggs, Enneagrams, and the thirty-eight Bach Flower typologies.

Given that we all have personality styles, some more conventional than others, the question naturally arises: What defines a certain personality style as dysfunctional or malfunctioning? The answer is not so easy.

In a personality disorder, the individual has a distorted, intensified, pathological expression of what might ordinarily be an average personality style. It is normal for a person to feel sadness or depression. When this state becomes chronic and inflexible to the point of affecting the individual's ability to function, this depression may be characterized as a personality disorder.

A person who can adjust to changing circumstances, is functional at his or her occupation, and has effective social skills might be said to have a healthy personality. Some individuals have unconventional personality styles. Some of these individuals may even become depressed because they do not easily fit into conventional patterns. An emotionally healthy but extremely unconventional personality has the ability to adapt just enough to function unconventionally in a conventional environment. People who are chronically depressed seem unable to adjust to a changing environment. The depressed person has deeply ingrained, enduring beliefs, rigid patterns of thinking, and behavior patterns that interfere with their ability to hold a job or socially interact. Some mental health professionals see these individuals as victims of a mental illness that needs to be treated with drugs. There is a thin line, therefore, between a personality disorder and an unconventional personality style.

Sometimes the Diagnosis Is Wrong

Many progressive thinkers in the mental health field question whether or not it is appropriate to automatically label what seems to be a personality disorder—especially depression—as a disease or illness. A disease label may make it easier for a physician to put a lot of symptoms into one basket, but the truth is that there are many types of depression, each type unique, and often a shifting group of symptoms. Is it effective or even fair to label individuals the victims of mental illness when what they are experiencing is an exaggerated variation or accentuation of one or more traits that make up a personality?

In the early days of mental health research, it was typical for psychiatrists and psychologists to diagnose individuals as mentally ill based on certain symptoms or personality patterns. Many psychologists question the appropriateness of this, since the medical model used to diagnose physical diseases does not apply as well to personality problems, which more often than not are particular types of problems in living. In 1995, M. A. Schwartz cowrote an article, "Prototypes, Ideal Types, and Personality Disorders: The Return to Classical Phenomenology." He quotes Kurt Schneider (1923), an early and seminal theorist of what is presently labeled personality disorders, on the inappropriateness of applying symptomology to personality:

> Psychopathic [i.e., personality] types look like diagnoses but the analogy is a false one. A depressive psychopath is simply a "certain sort of person." People or personalities cannot be labeled diagnostically like illness or like the psychic effects of illness. At most, we are simply emphasizing and indicating a set of individual peculiarities which distinguish these people and in which there is nothing compa-

rable to symptoms of illness. . . . In any detailed portrayal the type is soon lost and other traits not necessarily linked to the special characteristic in question creep in to form a concrete portrait. . . .[10]

Depression Is Often Underdiagnosed

Many experts say that depression is often underdiagnosed and untreated. An often overlooked aspect of undiagnosed depression is that it can become a complicating factor and unseen consequence of other seemingly unrelated diseases. Experts have reported that undiagnosed depression can seriously interfere with treatment and rehabilitation in many other physical and mental illnesses, including eating disorders and substance abuse.

The medical and mainstream mental health approach to depression is primarily a system of disease classification. Mental disorders are named primarily by the dominant symptoms they exhibit and not on biological or psychological processes. The flaw in this approach is that, though diagnosing depression is easier this way, it overlooks the more difficult reality that there may be a specific causative factor of a specific individual's depression that has not been isolated.

Many doctors are ignorant of how to address depression when it is a cofactor of other diseases. In fact, it is not uncommon for depression to be explained away, missed entirely, or masked by another disease. This happens so often that an individual considered a difficult patient with a bad attitude may, in fact, be suffering from depression.

To truly define *depression*, a physician must screen patients by asking them the appropriate questions. In 2002, the U.S. Preventive Services Task Force, an influential, independent panel of experts concerning United States healthcare policy, recommended that physicians screen all adult patients for depression. Based on a review of the published medical literature from January 1994 through August 2001, the task force discovered a 13 percent reduction in risk of chronic depression among screened individuals compared to those who were not screened. The task force also discovered that merely asking simple questions of the patients concerning the presence of depressive symptoms appeared to be as effective as longer, more comprehensive screening tools. The panel does not make suggestions for frequency of screening or for any specific approaches to treatment. Once this screening process is done and it is, in fact, determined that a person suffers from depression, the process still requires that the source or multiple sources of the depression be isolated. According to Norman Sussman, clinical professor of psychiatry at New York University School of Medicine, "Depression tends to be under-diagnosed—at least half of all depressions are not diagnosed right now."[11]

Proper diagnosis of clinical depression should include standardized techniques for assessing cognitive, behavioral, and emotional functioning, including neuropsychological and psychological tests, scales that rate behavior, and controlled interviews. Clinical neuropsychological assessment should be included to determine the course of an illness, to assess neurotoxic effects (for example, a memory deficit by substance abuse), to differentiate depression from dementia, to identify cognitive defects, to evaluate the effects of treatment (for example, surgery for epilepsy or psychopharmacology), and to evaluate learning disorders.

Brain Electrical Activity Mapping

Brain electrical activity mapping (BEAM) is a noninvasive, computerized testing method that analyzes the electrophysiological status of the brain. The one-hour-long BEAM process was developed at Harvard Medical School by Frank Duffy, M.D., in the late 1980s. It consists of five sets of measurement. The BEAM test allows physicians to address brain dysfunction in ways that were previously unavailable even with magnetic resonance imaging (MRI) or computed axial tomography (CAT) scanning.

BEAM can analyze many different functions of the brain by evaluating critical markers and correlating them to individuals suffering from various mental and emotional problems, including depression. BEAM tests can analyze how the brain receives and processes incoming stimuli. These measurements are electronically analyzed against normal parameters. The data collected through BEAM has been found to be clinically relevant to the study of depression.

In addition to screening for depression through an interview and questioning of a patient, a full head-to-toe physical evaluation should be conducted, including blood and urine analysis, to seek out biochemical causes of depression. Then a BEAM test should be done.

Eastern Diagnostic Approach

There are many diagnostic approaches that have been used in Asia and among aboriginal peoples throughout the world that do not fit the

Western scientific model. Traditional Chinese Medicine (TCM), like Indian Ayurveda, never separates the mind, body, and spirit. All these elements of the individual are addressed in both the diagnostic and the therapeutic process.

In TCM, a thorough diagnosis of the client is always conducted by means of an in-depth evaluation of the patient's symptoms and from the evaluation of energetic imbalances.

The perspective of Chinese medicine is to explore a wide-ranging configuration of symptoms. Various combinations of symptoms may indicate a unique pattern of disharmony, which requires different treatment approaches. It is difficult for a Western-based physician or scientist to understand this approach since meridians, tsubos, vibrational energy, yin yang, and chi are all concepts that are totally foreign to a Western biomedical, mechanistic approach to healing.

Unlike Western medicine, energetic or vibration medicine, whether Ayurvedic or TCM, has a treatment for every diagnosis.

Beginning the Healing Process

Unless there is a clear biochemical or electrophysiological factor causing the depression such as hypoglycemia, magnesium deficiency, chemical sensitivity, deficiency of sunlight (SAD), brain injury, or a brain chemical imbalance—diagnosing and defining treatment options for depression become a step-by-step, trial-and-error process. It is hard to know which approach or treatment will be most effective for each problem. The key is in recognizing that depression may be a factor in many seemingly unrelated conditions.

A truly integrated way of understanding the source and patterns of an individual's depression is through four key perspectives. These four perspectives need to be integrated in the evaluation of the client. They are:

1. The specific symptoms and their biochemical cause.
2. Psychological variation.
3. The client's behavior patterns.
4. The client's personal life history and background.

This is not so radical an approach since a variation of this system has been used at Johns Hopkins, a prestigious research center, university, and hospital since the late 1970s.

Once the depression is therapeutically addressed, there may be an immediate reduction of symptoms related to other medical and mental conditions. This then may lead to better patient cooperation and compliance concerning the treatment of these conditions. Conversely, as these medical disorders are more effectively treated, there may be a reduction in the symptoms of depression, and this may even result in the prevention of depression as a secondary disorder.

Physical-based illness and depression frequently occur together. In many cases, there is an absence of a demonstrable organic basis for either illness. There is then a great temptation to attribute the underlying causes purely to psychological factors, such as anxiety or stress. Conversely, like many physical illnesses, depression may be the end result of a complex series of bodily events culminating in neuropsychological activity.

For centuries, it has been known that physical illness can be relieved or modified by psychological means. However, only recently has any serious attention been given to the biochemical causes of depression. If psychological intervention can relieve a headache, can changes in body chemistry influence mood?

It should also be recognized that at least some of the depression found in patients with physical illness may be a secondary effect of the pain, distress, or disability caused by the physical illness. Not unexpectedly, when the physical illness clears, the patient experiences an elevation in mood. This clearing may be primarily psychological or it may be a response to chemical changes. The next chapter will address some of these issues.

2 🌹 THE BIOLOGY OF DEPRESSION

When examined closely, most depression manifests as a distortion of brain wave patterns and/or an imbalance in the biochemistry in the brain. These imbalances lead to emotional and psychological distortion and the resultant "ineffective thinking." Depression is often the end effect of a long interrelated chain including genetic predispositions combined with environmental influences and biochemical factors such as high levels of free radicals and heavy metals. Individually, these factors might not be that influential on an individual's emotional state, but combined, they could have a devastating effect. The general approach that Western physicians take to treat depression is increasingly antidepressant medication.

In this chapter we will examine the role of receptors in brain health, brain wave states, and the causative factors in depression.

Antidepressant Medication

People are often prescribed drugs to alleviate the symptoms of certain types of depression even when the depression might be best addressed by simply feeling and working through the emotion. Certain emotions need to be experienced as a healthy part of living, and medications interfere with this process. Are drugs, therefore, really necessary? For some people, the answer is yes. But no matter how effective medications are at the beginning, they do not correct ingrained character difficulties.

Short-term hospitalization may be necessary during times of extreme stress, impulsive behavior, suicidal patterns, or substance abuse. But for many individuals, long-term outpatient psychotherapy, biochemically based nutritional and herbal approaches, emotional healing, spiritual counseling, and group therapy in which the group vision and style match the clients' needs can be very helpful. Though some individuals respond dramatically to any of a number of natural approaches to deep-rooted chronic depression, more often than not, treatment is difficult and long-term. The symptoms of depression may often interfere with the therapy process. Periods of improvement may appear and suddenly be replaced with a worsening of some symptoms, but hope should never be lost. Over time, most people experience a great reduction in their depression and the associated symptoms of coexisting disorders.

In addition, since some types of depression do not respond to one drug, doctors may prescribe four or five different drugs. Even when medications can reduce and even control certain symptoms of depression, they are not a cure for the disease. Most severely depressed people who use drugs as their sole treatment risk further breakdowns.

Medications, in general, tend to be very complex in structure. So complex, in fact, that it is virtually impossible to know how any one drug might react with every other drug, food additive, and nutrient that it might come in contact with. For this reason, drugs should be used only when absolutely necessary, since the brain has tremendous difficulty metabolizing them.

"There is too often an unrecognized link between depression and other medical, mental and substance abuse disorders," said Dr. Rex W. Cowdry, acting director of the National Institute of Mental Health. "Co-occurring depression is common and can have a big impact on treatment and recovery, but many people, including doctors, are not addressing it as a serious problem."[1]

If you are taking any medications, know the side effects of every one and any interactions each drug may have with other medications, nutrients, or herbal products.

The Role of Receptors in Brain Health

The human brain, at about three pounds of tissue, is the most complex of our organs, playing a key role in the health of all other organs, glands, and bodily functions. The brain is the physical foundation from which thoughts, emotions, and feelings emanate, and a healthy brain creates the foundation for physical and emotional health.

One definition of health is a person's ability to communicate effectively. In addition to communication between people, there is also biological communication—the communication that takes place between different parts of your body. Your body is made up of millions of cells, and they have to be able to communicate with each other effectively. Part of how this takes place is through receptors.

A receptor essentially is a cellular tool whose purpose is to receive biological signals. Part of how each cell functions is that it has a receptor that receives specific signals and produces an appropriate response. Effective biological communication depends on various substances, including nutritional factors, immunotransmitters, peptides, and neurotransmitters. These substances influence the brain and the body on a cellular level. When the brain receives unbalanced levels of essential nutrients or toxic, heavy metals, serious problems can arise concerning neurotransmitter levels. This is especially so since heavy metals can replace essential nutrients (particularly minerals), fooling the brain and causing deficiencies. A neurotransmitter may even bind to a receptor in certain cells and set into action a complex series of events at a molecular level. These events may influence various brain functions including memory, mood, and behavior.

Brain Wave States

Researches have shown that certain processes—including emotional changes in the brain—produce measurable activity. This type of activity is known as brain waves. Brain waves can be measured (as cycles per second, called *hertz*), and an understanding of brain waves can be an important tool in addressing mental and emotional health issues. There are many levels of brain waves, but researchers divide them into four primary distinct varieties: beta, alpha, theta, and delta waves.

Many researchers are studying the distortions of brain wave patterns as a factor in mental illness, including depression. Techniques used to treat depression, including meditation, hypnosis, and aromatherapy, derive their effectiveness in part from their influence on these brain wave patterns. This is discussed in greater depth in Chapter 8.

Causative Factors in Depression

There are many different factors that can cause depression. Whatever the primary cause, the response of the brain to any of these is an altering of brain chemistry. In the following pages, we will discuss the more common factors.

The Neurotransmitter Factor

Some, though not all, depression seems to be connected in one way or another with specialized brain chemicals called neurotransmitters. There are over 100 different kinds of neurotransmitters. Of these, three seem to have the greatest influence on depression. These are norepinephrine, dopamine, and serotonin. These neurotransmitters, known as the *catecholamines*, follow pathways going deep into various parts of the brain (for example, the hypothalamus) that are responsible for the functions most commonly affected by depression—appetite, sexual interest, mood, and sleep.

Though researchers are not clear how direct the connection is, clearly catecholamine levels are related to depression, because the antidepressant drugs that specifically boost levels of these neurotransmitters also relieve depression.

Recent research indicates that there is much more involved in brain activity and depression than neurotransmitter levels alone. Many experts agree that depression is influenced by highly complex interactions of receptor responses (the ignition of action potentials) and the release of neurotransmitter "keys" (the keys that fit into specific receptors).

It also seems that depression levels depend on the quality and availability of the receptor "ignitions," not just on the number of neurotransmitter "keys." When there is a balance between ignition and keys, brain function is balanced. When the number of receptor "ignitions" is out of balance with transmitter "keys," depression may result.

Research indicates that when neurotransmitter levels are abnormally low, messages are unable to effectively cross synaptic gaps, resulting in a slowing down of communication in the brain. Many factors can contribute to the biochemical disruption in pathways responsible for serotonin and norepinephrine production and distribution, including the respective receptor sensitivities and inhibitory mechanisms in the function of the hypothalamus.

The only raw materials for the synthesis of neurotransmitters are nutrients, including amino acids, essential fatty acids, vitamins, minerals, and cholesterol. Deficiencies in any of these factors, or an abnormal intake of what are known as toxic heavy metals, may cause depression.

Depression can also result when brain neurotransmitters are unable to fit into the receptors for one reason or another, or if there aren't enough of these neurotransmitters circulating in the brain.

Estrogen Dominance

A cause of many health problems associated with PMS and menopause, including depression, hypoglycemia, and mood swings, is a condition known as *estrogen dominance*. This condition results when the normal ratio or balance of the hormones estrogen and progesterone is shifted by an excess of estrogen or inadequate amounts of progesterone. This problem and how to respond to it is discussed in greater depth in Chapter 5.

Electropollution

Electropollution is caused by excessive exposure to certain types of energetic frequencies such as the nonionizing electromagnetic radiation (NEMR) emitted primarily by radar installations, microwave appliances, and broadcast towers and by magnetic fields surrounding power lines and electrical appliances.

If you are depressed and you suspect the cause is electropollution, the solution is to reduce prolonged use of cellular and cordless phones and minimize prolonged proximity to working electrical appliances. Obviously it is almost impossible to completely avoid electronics, but you can be conscious and keep your distance when possible. Stay three or four feet away from your computer, leave the room if microwaving food, and keep eight to ten feet away from your television when it is on.

Genetic Factors

Though depression has been known to run in families, there is no evidence in the medical literature that "depression" is a genetic disorder. Attitudinal patterns, as well as nutritional and eating patterns, can pass from generation to generation, and these factors may influence certain biochemical and emotional factors that might contribute to the onset of depression.

Though there may not be a specific genetic marker for depression, some researchers believe that certain individuals may carry an inborn sensitivity to the disease that can be triggered by environmental factors, by changes in body chemistry, or by a psychological trauma. It is certainly possible that a strong genetic component might exist in an individual causing improper metabolism of certain nutrients, such as magnesium, chromium, or inositol—all nutrients essential for proper mental health.

One biochemical cause of depression is a genetic inability to manufacture enough of the important brain metabolite prostaglandin E1 (PGE1), which is derived from essential fatty acids. Individuals with this problem have a congenital deficiency of omega-6 essential fatty acid. Alcohol stimulates temporary production of PGE1 and lifts the depression. Sadly, this cycle may cause a depressed individual with this condition to abuse alcohol. Ultimately the resulting alcoholism can lead to other problems that aggravate the preexisting depression.

Any means of providing the brain with PGE1 can reverse depression and reduce the dependency on alcohol. Those who lack the ability to do this normally can correct this problem by taking a gamma-linolenic acid (GLA) supplement. Herbally derived evening primrose oil is a good source for GLA. Many nutritionists recommend that GLA be taken with zinc, vitamin B_6, and vitamin C. Zinc is needed for the formation of GLA; vitamin B_6 is important for the metabolism of cis-linolenic acid; and vitamin C is important to increase production of PGE1. Many people have claimed that this combination of four nutrients began to lift their depression in just a few days.

Another example of a hereditary biochemical abnormality that might contribute to the onset of depression is a genetic disorder involving a body chemical called pyrrole. Pyrrole is a simple chemical structure used by the body in the creation of heme, which makes blood red.

Pyrroles bind first with vitamin B_6 and then with zinc, depleting these essential nutrients. Since vitamin B_6 is an essential factor in the final steps of serotonin production, depletion of this nutrient might cause individuals who suffer from a genetically based pyrrole disorder to experience extreme mood swings.

Genetic predisposition, when combined with stress and stressful lifestyle patterns, can lead to biochemical imbalances. Biochemical imbalances, which may include clinical and subclinical nutritional deficiencies, can be aggravated in susceptible individuals by the intake or use of heavy metals such as lead and cadmium, addictive substances, alcohol, nicotine, and caffeine, as well as allergies or food sensitivities to corn, wheat, yeast, milk, or soy products. Nutritonal deficiencies can also be caused by the excessive use of refined foods. The result of all of these factors is an imbalance of hormones and blood sugar, all leading to depression and an increased and complex cycle of nutritional deficiencies aggravated by an increased use of refined food products and addictive substances. This destructive cycle increases the systemic damage, which leads to greater biochemical imbalances.

Imbalances in the Circadian Rhythm

The circadian rhythm is an inherent cycle, approximately twenty-four hours in length, that appears to control or initiate various biological processes, including wakefulness, sleep, and hormonal and digestive activity. A key, defining factor for depression in many people is their circadian rhythm and the relationship of this rhythm to the twenty-four-hour dark-light cycle. This dark-light cycle affects a multitude of bodily functions, including the output of melatonin and serotonin. A radical shift in any of these body functions might cause an altered emotional response, resulting in depression.

The natural signal for the circadian pattern is the shift from darkness to light. Exposure to bright natural or artificial light in the morning can help reestablish normal circadian rhythm and may increase hormone production, thus reducing depression.

Free Radicals

A key to healthy functioning of the brain is the relationship of brain cell membranes to antioxidants and oxidants. We all need oxygen, but even the most important biochemicals may be damaging when they appear in the wrong place, at the wrong time. For example, oxygen is essential for life, and yet when oxygen appears where it doesn't belong in the body, it can set off a chain reaction that ultimately results in the formation of molecular particles known as free radicals.

Free radicals are impossible to avoid just by eating healthier. They are created from elements in our external environment such as water and air pollution, dietary sources, and even certain medicines. Many of the problems we encounter with free radicals result when so many of them accumulate in our bodies that damage to the system results. Researchers have discovered that specific biochemical agents possess antioxidant properties. These nutrients, which include certain vitamins, minerals, amino acids, and substances found in some herbs, can reduce the negative effects of free radicals by reducing or stopping a harmful bodily process know as oxidation. Not all of these nutrients, known as antioxidants, are effective in the prevention of depression because they are incapable of entering the brain by passing through the blood-brain barrier. There are, however, lipid-soluble brain antioxidants that do reach their intended target in the brain and perform their tasks after moving from the circulatory system across the blood-brain barrier.

Some studies have shown that antioxidants can even help prevent the onset of certain neurological disorders. Different antioxidants are discussed further in Chapter 4.

Positive Ion Imbalances

In 1899, two scientists named Johann Elster and Hans Geitel proved the existence of ions, electrically charged particles in the air. The beneficial effect of some of these ions was initially discovered by Dr. C. W. Hansell at RCA Laboratories in 1932. Dr. Hansell was shocked and surprised by the extreme, violent mood shifts he observed in a coworker who was sitting next to an electrostatic generator. This same colleague seemed to become ebullient when the machine produced negative ions, and sad and depressed when it made positive ions.

Research conducted since the 1930s on ions has shown that positive ions generally have a negative effect on physical and emotional health. On the other hand, negative ions enhance physical and emotional functioning, stimulating everything from libido to plant growth.

A depressed individual should try as much as possible to be in an area with a greater level of negative-to-positive ions. This is not always easy, since many of those things that we most take for granted in our industrial society actually produce high levels of undesirable positive ions. A few of these positive ion sources include tire dust, heating and cooking fumes, car exhaust, factory fumes, and cigarette smoke.

Many other factors can actually absorb the desirable negative ions, thus creating an excess of positive ions. Among those things that can produce this undesirable effect include dust and soot, synthetic clothing and furniture coverings, synthetic building materials, metal ducts covering heating and air-conditioning outlets, and concrete and steel buildings. In a typical interior containing many of the materials listed above, the negative ion count may be extremely low.

Many physicians specializing in the treatment of depression now believe that increasing negative ion levels can promote our capacity to absorb and utilize oxygen, thus accelerating the blood's delivery of oxygen to our cells and tissues. Research also indicates that negative ions can increase alpha brain waves and brain wave amplitude, and reduce anxiety, neurosis, and depression. As a result of these clear benefits, they recommend negative ion–generating machines for suffering individuals. The development of safe and effective negative ion generators has been a long and complex process. Present ion units apply a high-voltage electrical signal directly to the air to create an intense electric field around the emitters.

Ionizers are now used throughout industry, and the U.S. government has even placed them in nuclear submarines. Designers and architects include waterfalls and fountains, which emit negative ions, in urban environments to bring the emotional benefits of nature indoors. Smaller, portable, individual models are inexpensive, car-friendly, and easily available.

The beneficial effects of negative ions are not permanent. Researchers point out that their effectiveness remains only as long as they're being inhaled.

If you decide to use a negative ionizer, keep the following in mind:

- If anything is between you and the ion generator, you will not receive the benefits of the ionizer.
- Dry indoor wintertime air may create a static charge that will often repel ions.
- Synthetic clothing absorbs ions. So wear natural fibers such as cotton or wool, which have neutral charges.
- Most machines produce one level of ion. However, there is a trend to measure and allow people to dial their needs electrically. Some European machines already modulate frequency.
- Although advanced technology has eliminated many problems associated with previous ion devices, the quality of machines still varies greatly.
- To guarantee that an ion-producing device meets your needs, carefully examine the manufacturer's literature. Purchase a product that offers a warranty on parts and labor, including a description of the room size affected by the machine.

Parasites

Many physicians and nutritionists believe that one of the most under-diagnosed and problematic causes of various illnesses, including depression, are parasitic infections. According to Dr. Hazel Parcells, an expert on parasitic "worms" (a type of parasite), they are the most toxic agents in the human body. "They are one of the primary underlying causes for diseases and are the most basic cause for a compromised immune system."[2]

A 1976 nationwide survey on the infestation of parasites, conducted by the U.S. Centers for Disease Control (CDC), showed that one in every six people selected at random in the United States was hosting at least one form of parasite. Over 130 different parasites are known to invade humans, ranging in size from microscopic, single-celled protozoans to the 36-inch-long tapeworm.

Louis Parish, M.D., a former investigator for the Department of Health and Human Services, Public Health Service, stated in a report he prepared for the Food and Drug Administration (FDA) that as much as 20 percent of the world's population is infected by protozoans. Through careful diagnosis, he also determined that at least eight out of ten of his patients had some variety of parasitic infections.

Parasites are able to travel almost anywhere in soft tissue, including the brain. Though the majority of infected individuals are symptom-free, persons with low resistance can find parasitic infections most destructive. In his report for the FDA, Dr. Parish further reported that, "Protozoal infection is accepted in most parts of the world as a way of life, just as we accept the common cold. It is, however, by no means limited to the tropical areas of the world. In fact, it has been shown that one out of four tourists to Leningrad become infected."[3]

One might think that, with the sophistication of healthcare in the United States and the huge amounts of money spent on public health education, parasitic infections would be a rarity rather than widespread. Yet there are a number of factors that have helped the spread of this condition, including:

- Increased mobility and travel for business and tourism, which have brought people to areas where there is infected food or water.
- Drinking tap water. It is believed that *Giardia lamblia* (a protozoan) has infected as much as 50 percent of the U.S. water sup-

ply and it is unaffected by chlorination. The presence of this parasite reduces the secretion of immunoglobulin A, thus depressing the effective functioning of the immune system.

• Use of antibiotics and other medications and chemicals that lower immunity.

• New patterns of sexuality whereby individuals come in contact with numerous sexual partners.

According to Dr. Parish, malnutrition can be caused by parasites leeching nutrients from their host. This can result in many of the symptoms associated with depression, including fatigue, as well as various digestive and immune disorders.

Parasites are hard to diagnose. The most widely used diagnostic test for parasites is random stool samples, and this approach has been found to be unreliable. Parasitic infections as a cause of various health problems are often ruled out on the basis of false negatives. Once parasitic infection is positively confirmed, the standard medical treatment for the infection is with chemical agents that produce strong side effects, in addition to weakening the already repressed immune response.

Grapefruit seed extract and olive leaf extract have been found to be very effective against a broad range of parasitic invaders. According to Dr. Parish, grapefruit seed extract, which he says does not cause side effects, "is as effective as any other amoebicide now available, perhaps more effective."[4] Dr. Parish and his associates treated nearly 200 patients for *Entamoeba histolytica* and *Giardia lamblia* over a two-month period. Dr. Parish went on to say how grapefruit seed extract "gives symptomatic relief more than any other treatment."[5]

Heavy Metals

Depression can result from heavy metal contamination of the body, especially with mercury, lead, copper, and aluminum. Those most vulnerable to this condition include those who have amalgam dental fillings, eat a lot of fish, drink water containing high heavy metal levels, do not properly wash their produce containing pesticides, or live in areas with air pollution problems. Toxic heavy metals can be screened for by way of hair analysis.

Some solutions to the heavy metal problem include:

- Avoidance of further exposure to heavy metals through the implementation of dietary and nutritional supplementation strategies. Chelation therapy can also remove these metals from the body. Meso-2,3-dimercaptosuccinic acid (DMSA) is a water-soluble, sulfhydryl-containing compound that is an effective oral chelator of heavy metals. Speak to your nutritionally trained, holistic physician about chelation therapy to remove toxic metals from your system.
- Zinc supplementation. It has been found that this can eliminate copper accumulation in the brain, thus eliminating the depression common to Wilson's disease patients.
- Use of magnesium as a calcium channel blocker. This is one solution to the problem of prescription calcium channel blockers.

Other physical-biomedical causes of depression can include calcium channel blockers (the prescribed remedy for Wilson's disease, a serious copper accumulation disease), endocrine abnormalities, connective tissue–collagen disorders (arthritis), drug side effects, viral disease, grief, cancer, vitamin B_{12} deficiency, anemia, folate deficiency, an organic brain disorder, fatigue, and chronic pain.

Chronic Fatigue Syndrome

Chronic fatigue syndrome (CFS) is an immune condition that may lead to depression. CFS is also known as chronic Epstein-Barr virus (CEBV) and chronic fatigue immune dysfunction syndrome (CFIDS). Outside of the United States, it is known as myalgic encephalomyelitis (ME). Many of the symptoms associated with this condition are evident in those suffering from chronic depression.

The symptoms of CFS are characterized by debilitating fatigue, experienced as exhaustion and extremely poor stamina (especially after a stressful activity or experience), neurological problems, mental fogginess, insomnia, and oftentimes, gastrointestinal problems. Numerous other symptoms will come and go and will vary among different patients. The severity of these symptoms will also vary over time for the same patient.

The cause of CFS is not yet known and it is extremely difficult to diagnose. Preliminary research indicates that it may involve a brain disorder that affects the body's stress response system, or causes an overactivity of the immune system.

Though there is no definitive way of diagnosing this condition, an effective laboratory diagnosis can be made on a single acute-phase serum sample by testing for antibodies to several CEBV-associated antigens simultaneously. In most cases, a distinction can be made as to whether a person is susceptible to CEBV, has had a recent infection, has had an infection in the past, or has a reactivated EBV infection.

There is no specific treatment for CFS. However, individual symptoms can be treated. The most promising method of treatment appears to be activating the immune system through a series of indirect methods. These methods include diet, high doses of vitamins and minerals, exercise and rest, affirmations, visual imagery, and positive thinking.

There are no prescription antiviral medications that are of proven or suspected value.

Bipolar Disorder

Bipolar disorder is a mental disorder distinguished by episodes of mania and depression. Until several years ago, it was more commonly known as manic depression.

There are a number of issues involved in bipolar disorder. Identifying and correcting them are important factors in healing this illness. The key issues are:

- Nutritional imbalances and subclinical deficiencies owing to an inability to manufacture enough stomach acid. The ability to produce adequate stomach acid is essential for the body to digest and absorb an adequate supply of essential nutrients.
- Candida overgrowth. This yeast condition is common among the psychiatric population in general, especially among those suffering from bipolar disorder.
- Parasites. Parasites, which may go unrecognized for decades, are more common than most people realize. They not only utilize nutrients from the system that are essential for good emotional health, but release toxins into the system as well.
- Nutritional imbalances and subclinical deficiencies owing to chronic and/or recurrent digestive enzyme deficiency. These biochemical imbalances may cause or indirectly influence erratic swings in blood sugar owing to hormonal imbalances and pancreatic insufficiency and overactivity resulting in hypoglycemia. A

deficiency of oxygen to the brain, which results from low blood sugar, can cause damage to essential body tissues—especially cerebral tissue. This damage to essential body tissues can create greater biochemical imbalances that may affect immunity and allow infectious invasions of various types to take place.

Bipolar individuals are often lacking in digestive enzymes. Since the production of these enzymes requires many of the same amino acids and minerals that are needed for the manufacturing of neurotransmitters, it is not unreasonable to assume that if a person lacks an adequate supply of digestive enzymes, they may lack neurotransmitters as well. This essential biochemical factor needs to be addressed in any person with any psychiatric diagnosis. One solution is to use pharmaceutical-grade digestive enzymes.

- Hidden allergies or sensitivities to foods or chemicals. These are common among the bipolar population. There is no single food allergy test accurate enough to determine conclusively that a hidden allergy is the cause of bipolar disorder. However, a combination of the various tests available—especially the "elimination system"—can point a person in the right direction.
- An imbalance in types of bowel flora. This problem is often related to candidiasis but not always. A pharmaceutical-grade probiotic supplement is essential for any individual suffering from a psychiatric illness. Often, effective measures are also needed to thoroughly remove a variety of undesirable bacteria from the digestive tract, including the intestines.
- Deficiencies or imbalances in specific nutrients, including magnesium, calcium, chromium, and especially the amino acid glutamine.

If you suffer from bipolar disorder and ever think of hurting yourself or have suicidal thoughts, you should always work with a holistic physician when reducing or going off all psychotropic medications. You should never suddenly stop taking these medications. If appropriate, you can slowly phase them out under strict medical supervision over a six- to twelve-week period.

Toxic Indoor Environments

If you have a healthy lifestyle and become clinically depressed, the possibility exists that you may have a chemical sensitivity and are reacting to certain environmental pollutants. While investigating the cause of your depression, pay attention to any new patterns. Be sure to keep a log of dates and particulars, and investigate the environment of your home or place of work.

Fumes from cleaning products; oil finishes and preservatives; polishes and some shellacs (acceptable shellac should contain quick evaporation alcohol as a solvent); spackles and adhesives; paints, primers, and thinners; household detergents; chemical softeners; and solvents might have a negative emotional effect if you are chemically sensitive. If you want to avoid inhalant chemicals, there are many nonallergic, nonpolluting products available, but you have to look for them.

In addition to eliminating undesirable chemicals from the home and office, there are many other things you can do to improve your environment. Of greatest importance is the circulation of clean air. In many companies, there is no circulation of clean air because the air vents have been closed off. This may be done in an overzealous effort to conserve energy. This stale air is commonly called "blue haze." When air is stale, workers will get drowsy and become less productive. In a Virginia bank, vents that had been sealed for two years were opened, and the "blue haze" problem and its effects disappeared as if by magic!

My eight antidotes for indoor pollution are:

1. Use an electromagnetic shield on your video display terminal to cut low-frequency magnetic field emissions by 98 percent. These shields are available for most computers.
2. Make sure your laser printer has a filter that removes the ozone it produces.
3. Don't buy furniture with foam cushions and upholstery unless the product is made without chlorofluorocarbons, which are used to inflate foam products yet destroy the earth's protective stratospheric ozone layer.
4. Use furniture made with water-based adhesives and finishes.
5. Choose natural fiber carpeting and upholstery over synthetics. The latter release volatile organic compounds into the air.
6. Fill your office with plants and flowers. Spider plants and plants with hairy leaves absorb air pollutants (such as formaldehyde), produce oxygen, and add color to ease your eyes. Chrysanthemums, azaleas, and Gerbera daisies are similarly helpful.
7. Ask your cleaning service to use nontoxic, natural cleaners.

8. Avoid the popular typewriter correction fluids, which contain harmful chemicals that can deplete the stratospheric ozone layer. Instead, try Saunders Opti correction fluid, a nontoxic correction fluid that won't dry out when the bottle is still half full. It even smells fruity!

Beginning the Healing of Depression

Biological problems, especially biochemical imbalances, can result in mood instability and poor impulse control. This may ultimately result in poor social interactive skills and troubled relationships. Emotional challenges and limitations in childhood psychological development—especially those associated with abuse, neglect, or poor parenting—can create personality and self-image problems.

Effectively diagnosing and determining the cause of depression are only the beginning. Antidepressant medications may be helpful for some but clearly they are often used when unnecessary, are overprescribed by physicians, take weeks to show any effect, and are associated with numerous unpleasant side effects. The most effective approach to alleviating depression is to try to isolate the underlying psychological, nutritional, toxicological, and/or lifestyle influences, and address them in ways that require the least effort. The goal is to use the approach that has the fewest side effects, and produces the longest-lasting results.

Mainstream approaches to the treatment of depression often end up being a combination of stress management classes, psychotherapy, and antidepressant medication.

There is a better way. It is a process of exploration, support, discovery, a sense of partial redemption from a dark place, and further exploration, support, and discovery. It is a generally slow and unsteady process on a rough road, but in the end, the new ideas about life, the new friends and support, and the new way of living that is born through the process make the journey worthwhile.

3 ❧ EMOTIONAL HEALING WITH HERBS

Herbs are known to possess powerful psychological and mood-altering properties. Certain herbs and herbal substances may influence nutritionally based glandular imbalances in the pancreas, thyroid, and thymus gland, thus reducing depression.

Many herbalists work with mild mood restoratives known as nervines. These herbs do not work rapidly like drugs, but rather in a slow, rejuvenating manner.

Some nervine herbs, such as skullcap, licorice, vervain, marjoram, balm, and lavender, are best used by those troubled with a depression linked with insomnia or physical pain. Other herbs, such as ginseng, basil, and sage, are more appropriate for those who suffer from the type of depression that leaves them in bed with mental and physical fatigue. Some herbal antidepressives such as yerba maté, damiana, and kava kava have a mild, stimulating quality that gives the suffering individual a greater sense of aliveness and vitality. St. John's wort contains a chemical named hypericin, which is a monoamine oxidase (MAO) inhibitor, similar to antidepressant drugs in that category.

In this chapter, we will review the herbs that can help reduce or heal depression. We will also discuss how to purchase herbs and how to use them.

Choosing the Best Herbs to Heal Depression

Purchasing herbs can sometimes be a tricky business. What's on the label of an herbal product may not always be accurate or specific enough.

Factors that have an impact on the therapeutic quality of the product include:

- The species and part(s) of the plant used.
- When and where the plant ingredients were harvested, and where they were processed (different countries, for example, can have different manufacturing standards).
- Whether the plant ingredients have been standardized, what aspect of the plant has been standardized, and to what extent.

Many herbal and nutritional products can have drug-like effects, and some can be harmful if used irresponsibly. This has created a situation where orthodox physicians—many of whom were opposed to herbs and nutritional therapy to begin with—now use this and the labeling issue as excuses to attack herbal and nutritional therapies in one sweep. This is sad and irresponsible.

Certain herbal supplements (and other dietary supplements) may have damaging health effects. They may be poorly manufactured and thus be contaminated with other herbs, pesticides, and heavy metals. Some products may even have dangerous interactions with prescription drugs. Most herb supplements have no side effects, however, and when side effects are present, they are generally fewer and less dangerous than those of many drugs used to reduce depression. Herbal and dietary supplements also have a much better record concerning dangerous interactions with other drugs.

As the therapeutic use of herbs has grown in the last few decades, research into why they are so effective has also increased. Whereas traditional clinical herbalists combined herbs in unique ways to create specific formulas for the individual, some naturopathic physicians, pharmaceutical researchers, and medical herbalists wanted a more specific standardized product.

The origin of herbal products being offered in the form of standardized extracts was initiated in 1992 when a European Guaranteed Potency law was passed. On one level, it was a breakthrough since it enabled medical doctors, chiropractors, and consumers with no formal training in herbs to use herbal products with greater ease and confidence. The general thinking of those supporting standardized products was that if the active constituent of an herb has been isolated, then the therapeutic value of that herb would be increased by guaranteeing that a specific amount of that active constituent was in the herbal product.

One of the complaints that both herbalists and many consumers have with standardization of herbs is that there is no universally accepted "standard" for the manufacture of these extracts. One company's manufacturing methods may vary so greatly from another's that they seem to have virtually nothing in common except for the name of the herb on the label. Why? Because each company may use a different marker by which to base the standardization process. Though standardized extracts offer some assurance of what is in an herbal product, fraud and deception are still possible.

When choosing an herbal approach for the treatment of depression, keep in mind that standardized extracts of herbs such as St John's wort may have much value, yet standardized herbs and other products have many shortcomings and should not be relied upon exclusively.

Here are some points that may be helpful if you or someone you know is considering the use of herbal and dietary supplements for the treatment of depression or any other medical condition:

- Avoid looking for a magic answer. Occasionally there may be one key herbal or nutritional factor involved with a health problem, but often a combination of approaches is what will bring the quickest and longest-lasting results.
- If you are considering or organizing an herbal or botanical treatment, talk with a mental health professional or healthcare professional with a knowledge of depression as well as nutrition and herbs. This is important for your safety and for the development of an integrated and comprehensive treatment plan.
- Become informed about products and their ingredients and what is known scientifically about them. Request information from the product manufacturer or distributor.
- Consult a qualified herbalist who understands both traditional herbs and standardization. For help in finding such an herbalist, contact the American Herbalists Guild at 770-751-6021.

Herbal and nutritional products also have unique risks associated with their use. The companies that manufacture or package herbal and nutritional products are prohibited from making health claims about their products. Consequently, they are not required to warn consumers of interactions or side effects associated with these products.

All herbs are not safe. Certain herbs like foxglove (where digitalis was originally discovered) as well as pennyroyal can cause severe reactions in certain people and may even be poisonous for others. The words *natural, organic,* and *herbal* do not necessarily mean "safe." Read labels on prescription drugs and let your holistic physician or herbalist know all the medications and herbs you are taking. Differing herbal approaches may have a varying range of effectiveness and may not work the same way with all people. Thus, it is important to use all herbs and nutrients responsibly and get a thorough diagnosis from a competent physician before using alternative approaches.

Herbs That Can Help Reduce or Heal Depression

Over the years, herbal folk medicines and modern science have often been portrayed as oppositional. Many doctors, unfamiliar with the current research on herbs and mental health, may attack herbal approaches to health and healing as unproven or dangerous without understanding why or how they work. Many consumers use herbs indiscriminately, treating them as if they are drugs and using them to replace drugs in ways that are totally inappropriate.

There is no one proper way to use herbs to heal depression. Herbal products come in many forms and work in many different ways. Some affect the vibrational body and are used in unique, culturally based applications that cannot be tested through traditional scientific studies. Others work through the sense of smell and affect people according to their individual associations.

Thousands of herbs have been through scientific screening programs and some of them have been found to contain compounds that are clinically effective at treating certain health problems. Following are a few that may reduce or heal depression.

St. John's Wort

St. John's wort (*Hypericum*) is the herb that has received the greatest attention in recent years as a natural treatment for depression. The herb was used in ancient Greece as a remedy for nervous complaints. Though some psychiatrists are still resistant to its use, numerous placebo-controlled, double-blind studies support the success of St. John's wort extracts for the treatment of patients with depression. The popularity of this herb has grown not only because of its effectiveness in reducing depression, but because it has fewer and less severe side effects than antidepressant drugs—many of which may interfere with memory, sleep, and cognitive function.

If St. John's wort does exert its antidepressant and mood-elevating effects by inhibiting the enzymes that break down the brain chemicals noradrenaline and serotonin (as some researchers believe), it would be similar to the mechanism by which monoamine oxidase inhibitor (MAOI) antidepressant drugs produce their effects.

There are at least ten pharmacologically active constituents found in the extract of St. John's wort, but researchers are most interested in hypericin and pseudohypericin. The exact mechanism that enables the herb to reduce anxiety and depression has not been isolated. However, recent research indicating that the action of hypericin is at alpha receptor sites, known to be involved in the role of MAO and 5-hydroxytryptophan (5-HTP) reuptake inhibitors (a metabolite of L-tryptophan in the synthesis of serotonin), supports the belief of many that the herb is both a sedating agent and a mood elevator. Some researchers suggest the most effective dosage to be one standardized, 300-milligram tablet three times daily in extract form combined with the herb gingko, which is an antioxidant. If St. John's wort is going to be of help, results should begin to appear within two to four weeks.

Caution: People taking the anticoagulant drug warfarin should consult with a physician or pharmacist familiar with depression and herbs before taking St. John's wort. St. John's wort interferes with warfarin by reducing its blood levels and effectiveness. Preliminary evidence also suggests that it carries a risk of serotonin syndrome. This condition results from St. John's wort interacting with selective serotonin reuptake inhibitor (SSRI) drugs, such as fluoxetine (Prozac), causing side effects such as flushing, mental confusion, sweating, and muscle twitching.

New research suggests that St. John's wort is generally considered safe. However, there have been occasional reports that some individuals have experienced mild fatigue, increased skin and eye sensitivity to sunlight, itching, gastrointestinal distress, and dizziness. St. John's wort is generally safe during pregnancy and lactation, but long-term studies are lacking.

Though the use of St. John's wort is generally free of side effects, some individuals using this herb may experience photosensitivity rashes when exposed to sunshine Also, allergic reactions may occur in individuals who generally experience allergies to herbs. St. John's wort should also not be taken with antidepressant drugs because side effects may occur.

Kava Kava

In recent years the herb kava kava (*Piper methysticum*) has been promoted with great interest as an effective treatment for stress and anxiety disorders, including depression. Kava, the term used for the shrub and the beverage made from its root, is found in Micronesia, Hawaii, Polynesia, Melanesia, and other Pacific Islands, where it has been used in ancient ceremonies. Traditionally, the root was ground to a brownish powder, then mixed with water and consumed as a beverage.

Most kava kava products sold in the United States contain about 30 percent kavalactones (the active constituents). Many medical studies, including one published in 1997 in the journal *Pharmacopsychiatry*,[1] have found kava kava to be useful in reducing stress and anxiety. However, recent evidence points to the possibility that kava kava may have damaging side effects for the liver.

Beginning in 2000, several reports from Europe indicated that a few individuals had experienced liver damage while regularly consuming kava kava. Similar reports concerning Americans have been reported in the media.

Until it is clear whether kava kava is a risk factor in liver disease, it is best to take the conservative approach. Kava kava has been banned in Germany and may be banned in Canada. If you presently use kava kava, it is best to reduce or stop your use of the herb. If you've been taking kava kava daily for more than a few months, you may wish to have a liver enzyme test. This is a simple blood test that is often done routinely as part of a blood analysis.

So much more can be said about the potential benefits of this herb, the active biochemical agents that make it work, and so on. However, knowing that there is even a slight chance that responsible use of this herb might cause liver damage, and knowing that there are many other ways, including herbal approaches, to healing depression, why take the risk until more is known?

The fact that a particular herb may present side effects is no reason to avoid using herbs. "Properly prescribed" drugs kill more people every year that any herb might. These medicines were the fourth leading cause of death in the United States in 1998, according to the *Journal of the American Medical Association.*[2]

Here is a simple herbal formula for reducing the effect of stress on your system. This formula reduces mental overactivity, induces sleep, and will help you relax. It is also a popular remedy for insomnia and disturbed sleep patterns. Add the following herbs (in liquid extract form) in equal parts to a six-ounce glass of water and take it three times a day: valerian, passiflora, vervain, skullcap, motherwort, cowslip, and lady's slipper.

Gotu Kola

Gotu kola (*Centella asiatica*) is a popular tropical plant that has been used in Ayurveda for the prevention of mental fatigue and enhanced con-centration and memory. Gotu kola is caffeine-free and has no relation to the kola nut that is used to make soft drinks. This nervous system stimu-lant is considered valuable in energetic-vibrational medicine and as one of the most spiritual and rejuvenating of herbs. It is said to fortify the im-mune system, to strengthen the adrenals, help overcome insomnia, and assist in calming the system during meditation. Recent studies indicate that gotu kola has a positive effect on the circulatory system to the brain by improving the flow of blood throughout the body and by strengthening the veins and capillaries. This can be invaluable for individuals who are inactive or confined to bed due to illness.

Gota kola is often used in combination with ashwaganda and shilajit for energy support. Another valuable herb is skullcap (*Scutellaria laterifo-lia*), which helps to calm and relieve an overly sensitized nervous system, and verbena (*Verbena officinalis*), an ancient herb used to relieve contin-uing sadness and unhappiness. These work nicely with gotu kola.

Shilajit

Shilajit is a little known and unusual natural product that may be helpful in rebuilding the health of a chronically depressed person. This substance is an exudate that is pressed out from layers of rock in certain mountains of high altitude, especially the mountains of Nepal. It consists of humus and organic plant material that has been compressed by layers of rock. Its humus content is formed when soil microorganisms decom-pose animal and plant material into elements usable by plants.

Shilajit has been used for thousands of years for many different health problems. It is listed as a healing agent in ancient Sanskrit writings and is used today in Ayurvedic health practices. The primary active ingredients in shilajit are fulvic acids, dibenzo alpha pyrones, humins, humic acids, and trace minerals.

According to Dr. Michael Hartman, an authority on shilajit, "Dibenzo Alpha Pyrones are able to pass the blood brain barrier and act as a powerful antioxidant protecting the brain and nerve tissue from free radical damage. It also inhibits the enzyme Acetylcholinesterase, which breaks down Acetylcholine. This will increase the levels of Acetylcholine." Low levels of acetylcholine are associated with Alzheimer's disease and poor memory and concentration. It is believed that the health benefits of shilajit are, in part, based on the ability of fulvic acids to transport the dibenzo alpha pyrones and trace minerals into the body.

The recommended amount for general use and to maintain optimal health is around 150 to 250 milligrams twice per day. Be sure to drink six to eight glasses of water per day. There is approximately a six-to-eight-week period for the therapeutic effects to be noticed. Shilajit is metabolized slowly, reaching maximum blood levels in twelve to fourteen hours. Though there do not seem to be any damaging side effects, some individuals report that, in the early stages of use, they have experienced loose stools or mild diarrhea, fatigue, headaches, and skin rashes. If this happens, decrease the dosage (number of capsules) until the symptoms go away, then gradually increase the dosage again.

Shilajit should not be used by those who suffer from hypoglycemia because it possesses a strong ability to lower blood sugar. Diabetics should monitor their insulin usage to prevent hypoglycemia. Shilajit also contains a very small amount of phenylalanine. Persons with phenylketonuria (PKU) should be aware of this.

Ashwagandha

The roots of the ashwagandha (*Withania somnifera*) shrub, which is now cultivated in India and North America, have been used in Ayurvedic medicine for thousands of years—particularly to promote sexual vitality. Researchers from Banaras Hindu University in Varanasi, India, have discovered that some of the chemicals within ashwagandha are powerful antioxidants and may influence brain chemistry. The antioxidant effect of active principles of this plant may explain the reported cognition-facilitating, antistress, antiaging, and anti-inflammatory effects. Ashwagandha is traditionally used in India to treat mental deficits, including amnesia in geriatric patients.

A study done in 1991 at the Department of Pharmacology, University of Texas Health Science Center, indicated that extracts of ashwagandha had gamma-aminobutyric acid (GABA)–like activity. This may account for this herb's antianxiety effects. Anecdotal reports suggest that ashwagandha may be helpful in reducing slow metabolism, fatigue, and depression without any significant side effects.

Bacopa Monnieri

Bacopa monnieri is a traditional South Indian herb that has become popular in the United States owing to the increased awareness of Ayurvedic medicine. Initially, bacopa became popular for the treatment of certain types of attention deficit disorder (ADD). Recent studies indicate that this herb inhibits serotonin reuptake, a similar action to that which Prozac creates. Bacopa is an overall nervous system balancer and thus its rejuvenative action is not limited to its influence on serotonin. Many herbalists combine bacopa with other nervous system rejuvenators, such as ashwaganda, ginko biloba, gotu kola, and covolvulvus pleuricaulis.

Chinese and Hawaiian Herbal Medicine

There are a number of Chinese herbs and mushrooms that have been found to balance the emotions and reduce the symptom of depression. They include cortex albizzia julbrissin, gingko biloba, and noni.

Cortex Albizzia Julbrissin

Cortex albizzia julbrissin (mimosa tree bark) is used by many TCM practitioners as an alternative to Prozac. It is traditionally used to relax and relieve emotional imbalances, especially when bad temper, depression, insomnia, irritability, and poor memory are present. The flower of the mimosa tree is used to relieve constrained liver chi, which is important to body detoxification and to calming the spirit when the associated symptoms of insomnia, poor memory, and irritability are present. Research has shown that the flower of the mimosa tree has a sedative effect.

Gingko biloba

Ginkgo biloba is a tree native to China that has been used therapeutically and medicinally for centuries. It not only improves circulation and oxygen supply to the brain, as well as protecting it from free radical damage, but also improves alertness by increasing the brain's alpha wave rhythms.

Preliminary research indicates that ginkgo has been shown to have an MAO-inhibitor action. This action reduces the breakdown of serotonin, thus enhancing the effects associated with dietary consumption of 5-HTP.

Other popular herbs in Chinese medicine for the treatment of depression include chamomile, damiana, graviola, maracuja, muira puama, mulungu, tayuya, una de gato, and covolvulvus pleuricaulis.

Noni

Noni (*Morinda citrifolia*) is a small evergreen tree found growing in open coastal regions, especially in the Pacific Islands at sea level, as well as in forested areas up to 1,300 feet. The plant, which is prized for its fruit, grows abundantly along lava flows in Hawaii. Noni fruit turns yellow as it ripens and naturally has a strong pungent odor and taste. When I have the opportunity to teach in Hawaii, my herbalist friends bring me noni vinegar, which contains the plant's medicinal properties. It is prepared by placing the fruit in a jar and letting it ferment naturally.

Though noni was a part of traditional Hawaiian healing, Western researchers developed an interest in the plant in 1957 when Ralph Heinicke, Ph.D., isolated an alkaloid in healthy human cells called *xeronine*. Xeronine converts certain brain proteins into active receptor sites for endorphins, the "well-being hormones." When the body's cells are deficient in xeronine, major health problems, including depression, may arise. Dr. Heinicke's research on noni began in 1950 and continued to1986. During this period, he discovered that xeronine and its precursor, proxeronine, are present in the noni fruit and become biochemically active when digested. It is believed that noni fruit may contain the inactive form of the enzyme needed to release xeronine from proxeronine.

Many herbalists recommend noni for its ability to ease anxiety and depression. These dramatic results may stem from noni's enhancement of immune and glandular function, especially through its influence on the pineal, thyroid, and thymus glands. It is believed that serotonin is produced and melatonin is synthesized in these three glands. Melatonin helps regulate sleep, mood, and ovarian cycles—all factors in depression. Noni also balances the body's pH levels, which affect one's ability to absorb minerals and vitamins.

Noni may also help reduce depression by improving certain body functions that have been shown to affect the symptoms of depression including poor digestion, drug addictions, and chemical sensitivity. Neuroscientists have recently discovered an important role antioxidants play in the central nervous system, and there are a number of herbal antioxidants that can be of help.

Intestinal Detoxification

The body is like a river. When it is clean, it is clear and full of life. When polluted, it is clogged and stagnant and everything connected to it is affected the same way. Cleansing the body's internal ecosystem—especially the liver—of toxic metabolic wastes and other clogging substances creates a new vibrancy. This vibrancy allows nourishment to enter the circulatory system, reach the glands and organs, and feed the brain with oxygen and other essential factors so that they can do their jobs properly. This promotes physical and mental homeostasis, and the body and mind's innate ability to keep itself in balance.

Digestive disorders are also part of the cycle that can lead to depression. When digestive function is inadequate, excessive gases form, creating pressure on the various organs, including the lungs. This pressure reduces the oxygen supply to the tissues, raising the carbon dioxide levels and causing general depression.

Certain herbs, including ginger, peppermint, raspberry leaf, lemon balm, and cloves, have a direct healing and cleansing effect on the organs involved in digestion. Intestinal cleansing with herbs is one of the most important elements of good emotional health. Herbal intestinal detoxification is a safe, gentle, and effective colon cleanser and intestinal regulator that flushes the lymphatic system, destroys the intestinal parasites that might be affecting normal brain function, and nourishes the endocrine system. It also acts as a powerful liver cleanser.

Here is an effective herbal formula for reducing depression: St. John's wort, rosemary, oats, Siberian ginseng, lavender, and gotu kola. Purchase these herbs as liquid extracts, mix equal parts as directed, and take with distilled water three times a day. These herbs serve as antidepressants and nerve relaxants.

Blood Cleansing

An important aspect of body purification is the "blood cleanse." This requires a combination of herbs that detoxify the blood and lymph as well as supporting liver function and optimal circulation. The Ayurvedic herbs known as manjistha and neem, combined with turmeric and burdock root, form an excellent detoxifying formula. Manjistha is a lymph and blood cleanser, neem is an antiseptic, turmeric is an anti-inflammatory and blood-purifying agent, and burdock root is an effective liver cleanser.

A classic Western herbal formula for assisting the body in the removal of trapped metals, chemicals, and drug residues is bugleweed, yellow dock, buckthorn bark, lobelia, and cilantro. Buy them as extracts. Place 20 drops of each in a glass of distilled water and drink three times a day.

Lymphatic Detoxification

The East Indian guggul family of herbs is popular in programs focused on detoxifying the deep tissues of the body. Guggul is often combined with kanchanar to detoxify the lymphatic system as well as balance the hormonal system, specifically the thyroid gland. Other herbal remedies traditionally used for lymphatic detoxification include chamomile, damiana, graviola, maracuja, muira puama, mulungu, and tayuya.

If you are pregnant, lactating. or under a doctor's care for any health condition, you should consult with your physician before taking guggul or any other supplement.

Herbal traditions have existed for more than 3,500 years, and with increasing discoveries of important herbal constituents, the role of plants in healing is growing in importance. Even so, research over the last few years has indicated more than ever that faulty nutrition is the source of many diseases, including certain types of depression. This being the case, it is essential than any herbal healing program for depression include an investigation into nutritional factors that may be playing a part. Even mild nutritional imbalances can lead to food sensitivity, glandular imbalances, and other chemical changes in the body that through a chain of events can lead to depression. In the next chapter, we will discuss how a whole-food nutrition program, proper balancing of the essential nutrients, effective nutritional supplementation, and other key nutritional variables can lay a foundation for preventing depression or healing it.

4 🗝 NUTRITIONAL FACTORS AND DEPRESSION

Among the hundreds—even thousands—of important chemicals found in our food, and the more than 3,000 additives used in the manufacturing and processing of our food, there are only six nutritional factors that are considered to be "essential" for life. By essential, we mean that these factors are required in the diet—that is, if you do not get the required minimum of each of these six nutrients in your diet, you may begin to experience both physical illness and radical changes in mood and behavior.

A deficiency of these essential nutrients can interfere with the production of brain chemicals, especially dopamine and serotonin, which are essential for emotional health. A deficiency of these two neurotransmitters will cause you to feel emotionally uneasy, and can lead to depression and other symptoms. If nutritional deficiencies are not corrected, they can lead to more extreme nutritional deficiency diseases, and even death. For instance, there are many anecdotal reports and a few studies indicating that supplementation with magnesium, essential fatty acids, and vitamins C and B-complex can reduce the number and level of bipolar disorder episodes.

The six essential nutrients are protein, fats, carbohydrates, vitamins, minerals, and water. The right combination of these essential nutrients can prevent, reduce, and even successfully eliminate various behavioral and emotional imbalances, including depression, bipolar disorder, attention deficit hyperactivity disorder (ADHD), learning disabilities, and various eating disorders. On the other hand, nutritional imbalances can lead to these very same conditions.

Research has shown that emotional health is strongly related to glandular function, and glandular function is strongly related to nutritional health. Some scientists believe that there is also a link between brain function and nutrient malabsorption. Statistics indicate that there is an increased incidence of depression in chronic digestive disorders such as celiac disease, and even in children who suffer from inflammatory bowel disease. This may trigger brain chemical imbalances directly linked with depression.

Studies have shown that various nutritional deficiencies—for example, of vitamin B_{12}, zinc, the amino acid tyrosine, essential fatty acids, chromium, iron, magnesium, and manganese—can contribute to depression and reduced mental performance either directly or through nutritionally based conditions such as hypoglycemia and chronic fatigue syndrome. Dietary management and nutritional approaches seldom have side effects and can usually be safely combined with medication once the latter is necessary.

In this chapter, we will discuss how nutritional deficiencies can be a cause of depression and how nutritional supplementation may help to relieve or even eliminate it.

Nutritional Deficiencies as a Cause of Depression

Many researchers into depression believe that among the key factors for the increase of this condition is the increased used of certain modern agricultural methods that have reduced or detrimentally altered the levels of certain nutrients in the American diet. These practices can influence emotional behavior and mood by:

- Inhibiting interleukin-6 (IL-6), which can cause anxiety and depression.
- Inhibiting cortisol, which can cause anxiety and depression.
- Increasing levels of serotonin, by acting as a serotonin reuptake inhibitor.
- Increasing MAO-inhibiting properties.

Among the nutritional factors that may influence one or more of these factors are the influence of magnesium, boron, and inositol levels on the decrease in the ratio of omega-3 to omega-6 fatty acids. Chronic stress has been found to alter the complex biochemical activity of the brain by interfering with the subtle balance of neurotransmitters. It also leads to the depletion of magnesium. Low magnesium levels have been implicated as a cause of depression.

Another factor is the effect of low levels of protein, B vitamins, and various antistress nutrients as a cause of impaired brain function.

Depressed patients may have disturbances in folic acid metabolism related to vitamin B_6, vitamin B_{12}, magnesium, or zinc deficiency, as well as other nutritionally influenced metabolic imbalances. With improvement in dietary supplementation and treatment of these deficiencies, depression can often be alleviated.

Potassium deficiency can negatively affect magnesium metabolism. People who do not use mineral supplements and do not regularly eat bananas and potatoes or Morton's Lite Salt can experience such an imbalance. Morton's Lite Salt is a balanced combination of sodium chloride and potassium chloride.

Excess intake of table salt (sodium chloride) or the ingestion of salty foods can disrupt potassium and magnesium balance, resulting in lower magnesium levels. In addition to other health problems, this can affect neurotransmitter levels, resulting in depression.

The misuse of diuretics drugs (water pills) to reduce water retention associated with PMS can lead to potassium deficiency, causing an imbalance in magnesium levels, which can manifest as depression.

Healing Emotional Problems Through Diet

It has become commonplace in recent years for some nutritionists to defend the moderate use of processed, denatured foods. Unfortunately, processed and refined foods can seldom be eaten as part of a balanced diet. Despite this, "fast," highly processed foods have become an essential part of the modern diet—so much so that these foods are served in public schools and hospitals as dietary mainstays.

The regular use of processed foods can influence both physical and emotional health because they are rich in refined carbohydrates and deficient in—even devoid of—essential nutrients. Emotional health is based on some level on a regeneration and normalization of endocrine function and glandular balance. These cannot be easily achieved without paying attention to the acid-alkaline balance, enzyme content, and freshness of the diet.

A well-balanced nutrition program can serve as a strong foundation for healing depression. In the following pages, we will review the essential elements of such a program.

Protein

Protein is the nutrient essential for building healthy tissue. Amino acids are the building blocks of protein and thus are found in all protein foods.

The typical American diet is rich in beef, chicken, whole milk products, and eggs. All of these have plenty of protein, but they may also be laden with pesticides, hormones, saturated fats, and various body-polluting substances. These are just the things we are trying to eliminate from the system since they may contribute to various food sensitivities and other health problems. One of the best ways to obtain high-quality protein without the body-polluting factors and the food sensitivity factor is to eat combinations of whole grains and beans—especially gluten-free grains such as rice and corn—as well as fermented dairy products such as yogurt, kefir, and buttermilk.

Generally speaking, to achieve emotional health, it is best to eat approximately 50 to 80 grams of protein per day. In place of all that red meat and animal protein, we now know that combinations of various vegetarian foods are a much healthier choice.

Essential Fatty Acids

As was mentioned in Chapter 2, your body's cells communicate with each other through receptors. Cell membrane receptors in the central nervous system are composed of many substances, including proteins and lipids (fats). The human brain is more than 60 percent structural fat, much of which is made from omega-3 fatty acids.

Research has shown that modification of the lipid content in older brains will affect the functionality of a receptor. This relationship between receptor function and lipid composition is called *fluidity*. The greater the fluid content in a cell membrane, the greater the biological effect will occur.

Fluidity of cell membranes is directly affected by diet. The more saturated fat you eat, such as those found in meat, chicken, whole milk products, and hydrogenated vegetable oils, the less fluidity there will be in your cell membrane receptors. This lowered fluidity will reduce the ability of your cell membrane receptors to receive specific messages to carry out biological communication. Many researchers believe that there is a close link between cell membrane fluidity, dietary fat, and neurological and psychiatric conditions, especially depression. With greater amounts of saturated fat in our diet, our receptors are less likely to respond effectively to neurotransmitters such as dopamine and serotonin.

Diets that are rich in unsaturated fats, particularly the omega-3 fatty acids, seem to reduce some types of depression. However, unsaturated oils are not the best choices. Sunflower oil, soybean oil, safflower oil, and most other vegetable oils contain lots of undesirable omega-6 fatty acids.

The dopamine and serotonin receptors of your brain are composed of omega-3 fatty acids, including DHA, eicosapentaenoic acid (EPA), and eicosanoids. The body does not have to get these directly from food sources since it can manufacture all of them provided there is an ample supply of the primary omega-3 fatty acid and alpha-linolenic acid (ALA). ALA can be found in various foods including canola oil, flaxseed, Brazil nuts, and green leafy vegetables.

Changing eating habits have increased the use of man-made fats known as trans-fatty acids. These saturated fats and vegetable oils are high in omega-6 fatty acids, and all interfere with our body's attempt to utilize the tiny amount of omega-3 fats (including DHA) that it gets in the typical diet. One of the causes of depression seems to be the result of a nutritional chain reaction that begins with the increased use of these undesirable types of fat.

If a person has a deficiency of DHA in their blood, their body may begin to use man-made trans-fat molecules as a construction material instead. Unfortunately, trans-fats (hydrogenated oils) have a different shape than DHA. The trans-fat causes the dopamine receptor to become deformed and it becomes dysfunctional. This dysfunctionality, over time, can result in learning and mood disorders, including depression. This situation is even more problematic for a child whose brain is still developing. Deficiencies of DHA have been implicated in various learning and behavioral disorders in children, including ADHD.

One way to balance omega-3 levels is to avoid any products containing trans-fatty acids. This would include any food that has oils that have been partly hydrogenated, partly hardened, or hydrogenated. These processed oils and fats are in the majority of prepared foods, including crackers, muffins, mayonnaise, French fries, doughnuts, breads, margarine, potato chips, and cookies.

The body uses the same enzymes to break down omega-3 and omega-6 fatty acids into various compounds. If high levels of omega-6 fatty acids and low levels of omega-3 fatty acids are in the bloodstream, these enzymes will most likely be used up by the omega-6 fatty acids, resulting in the inability of the body to manufacture DHA out of ALA.

The key then is to create a balance between these two fatty acids. In the United States, where an unbalanced diet is par for the course, the typical ratio is twenty-two to one in favor of the omega-6 fatty acids. A healthy ratio is between one to one and four to one.

Good nutrition for brain health should begin at birth. Studies have shown that infants who are fed formula in the United States receive almost no omega-3s. Omega-3 fatty acids are highly unsaturated essential nutrients that are an essential part of the neuronal cell membranes. Conversely, breast milk contains DHA, and if the mother's diet is healthy and rich in these fatty acids, her breast milk will be rich in them as well. Researchers have found that infants who are fed formulas enriched with omega-3s or who are breast-fed do better both visually and intellectually.

Thus, if a mother cannot breast-feed, it is important that any formula she chooses be rich in omega-3 fatty acids. Numerous epidemiological studies have been published demonstrating that a deficiency of omega-3 fatty acids may encourage the onset of depression, and that an adequate intake of these nutrients can contribute to the prevention of the disorder. Interestingly, this discovery was made when two researchers, J. R. Hibbeln and N. Salem Jr., noticed a number of publications that pointed out that many cholesterol-lowering programs lead to cases of depression and suicide. According to Hibbeln and Salem, these extreme emotional reactions were not based on the lower cholesterol level—as might have initially been thought—but rather on the fact that cholesterol-reducing diets often create a reduced dietary ratio of omega-3 to omega-6 fatty acids. This results in a lowering of the omega-3 fatty acid concentration in body tissues, and an associated reduction (at the same time) of DHA in the brain. It is Hibbeln and Salem's contention that if omega-3 fatty acid is replaced by omega-6 fatty acid, changes in neuronal cell membrane properties may occur, which will increase the vulnerability to depression.[1]

A good resource for fatty acid deficiency and health-related problems is the book *Essential Fatty Acids and Immunity in Mental Health* by

Charles Bates, Ph.D. In it, he offers a checklist of indicators that can give you the clues as to whether you may have an essential fatty acid deficiency. These include chronic depression; SAD; alcohol abuse; a family history of alcoholism, depression, schizophrenia, suicide, or other mental illness; a personal or family history of atopic eczema, cystic fibrosis, Crohn's disease, hepatic cirrhosis or Sjogren-Larsson syndrome, ulcerative colitis, irritable bowel syndrome, PMS, scleroderma, diabetes, or benign breast disease. Individuals of Native American, Irish, Celtic, Scottish, Welsh, or Scandinavian ancestry have an increased risk. Another sign is getting a lift from EFA-rich foods such as flaxseed, fish oil, or borage oil.[2]

Complex Carbohydrates

Carbohydrates, in their complex form, are essential for purification and rejuvenation. In addition to providing energy, many carbohydrate-rich foods supply significant amounts of minerals, B vitamins, and even protein—all of which are essential for emotional health and healing. Complex carbohydrates also help detoxify the body by converting certain chemicals, bacterial toxins, and some normal metabolites (the end-products of the physical and chemical processes involved in the maintenance of life) into a form that can be easily eliminated as waste.

Complex carbohydrate foods include beans, peas, nuts, seeds, vegetables, and whole-grain breads, cereals, and pasta. Starches—the best form of carbohydrates—include whole grains such as brown rice, millet, buckwheat (also known as kasha), and barley; along with beans and root vegetables such as potatoes, carrots, and yams. In the application of the Emotional Healing Program, presented in Chapter 11, you will want to add an increasing variety of these cleansing, energy-packed, mineral-rich foods to your daily diet. Be sure to avoid white rice, prepared cereals, and refined white flour products such as macaroni, white bread, and crackers.

Research has shown consistently that there is a direct relationship between food and certain types of depression. Clinical studies have shown that even small, subclinical deficiencies in essential nutrients can trigger episodes of depression. Carbohydrates are important mood regulators. Some people crave carbohydrates—especially pasta, sweets, and starches—and may find them stimulating or sedating. Nutrition researchers are not sure why these foods have this effect. However, many think it has to do with the *glycemic index* (a ranking system that indicates how quickly foods are converted into blood sugar).

Changes in dietary habits and intensive nutrient therapy have helped many people who suffer from depression, even those who did not respond to traditional psychotherapy or antidepressant therapy. Even healthy individuals have discovered that their psychological state has improved with better nutrition and certain nutritional supplements.

B Vitamins

The B-complex vitamins are key to mental and emotional health. Because the body cannot store them, we depend entirely on our daily diet to supply them. B vitamins are destroyed by caffeine, nicotine, alcohol, and refined sugars. Sadly, these are the substances that are most often consumed by alcoholics, almost to the exclusion of well-balanced high-nutrition foods. This B-vitamin deficiency resulting from substance abuse (yes, a depressed person often uses alcohol and coffee, smokes, is self-medicating, and abuses the medication to boot) can be a direct cause of depression.

A 1982 *British Journal of Psychiatry* article reported that 1 out of 172 successive patients admitted to a British psychiatric hospital for treatment of depression suffered most from a vitamin B_2 deficiency.

The B vitamins are found in grains including whole wheat, rice, corn, and buckwheat (buckwheat is actually a fruit, though it is used as a grain). Vitamin B_{12} is found in enriched yeast, dairy products, and other animal products.

Antioxidants

Many brain disorders and their behavioral symptoms may be caused by oxidation damage to the body. Symptoms include confusion and memory loss, as well as the irritability that some elderly people exhibit, which may result from atheromatous plaques forming on the inside of the brain arteries. Some studies have shown that antioxidants can help prevent the onset of certain neurological disorders.

Antioxidant properties may be found in herbs, vitamins, minerals, amino acids, phospholipids, and other nutritional factors, including algae such as spirulina and blue-green algae. Herbal antioxidants include turmeric, certain pine bark derivatives, and grapeseed extract. Among the most commonly recommended antioxidants are alpha-lipoic acid, L-glutathione, coenzyme Q10 (CoQ10), lecithin, superoxide dismutase (SOD), tocotrienols, selenium, L-glutamine, chromium, vanadium, L-tyrosine, lycopene, and vitamins A, C, and E. Recent research indicates that green tea, both as a beverage and an extract, is one of the most effective antioxidant agents.

After water, green tea is the second most consumed beverage in the world. In TCM, green tea has been recommended for headaches, which often accompany depression, general toxicity, immune system dysfunction, and a variety of other ailments. The green tea with the greatest medicinal properties is the unfermented variety, not the familiar green tea that goes through a fermentation process to create its taste, color, and aroma. Studies on the antioxidant capacity of tea showed that the antioxidant activity in dry tea exceeds that of twenty-two fruits and vegetables. This may be due to the tea's L-theanine content.

Water

Water is something that many of us take for granted. But it is the magic ingredient to the maintenance of life. The purifying benefits of water include cleansing the internal organs and moving nutrients throughout the system. In addition, water helps to maintain body temperature and to eliminate toxins from the bloodstream. Important to dieters, it also helps reduce hunger.

The following are the best methods for purifying water:

- Distillation. Water is vaporized then condensed, leaving behind the dissolved minerals. You can purchase distillers as portable units or buy steam-distilled water in most food markets.
- Deionization or charcoal purification. Water is passed through resins, which remove most of the dissolved minerals.
- Reverse osmosis. Water is forced under pressure through membranes, which remove almost all of the dissolved minerals.

Do not drink tap water. You are also better off avoiding bottled spring water, which is often contaminated due to inadequate testing and purity standards.[3]

Nutritional Factors and Brain Chemistry

Of all the cells of your body, it is your brain cells that are among the most sensitive to nutritional deficiencies. The simple sugar glucose is the brain's main source of fuel. When poor diet and glandular imbalances cause glucose levels to drop, poor neurological signal transmission results and a host of different emotional symptoms may arise, including mood swings, memory loss, and depression. Even slight nutritional deficiencies have been found to impair brain function.

There is a growing body of research that shows that a sudden shock, a life-challenging event, and general psychological stress can deplete tissue of certain chemicals essential for health functioning. Usually these deficiencies or imbalances involve coenzymes, vitamins, minerals, or hormones. These imbalances can cause symptoms of physical and mental illness, especially depression. A stressor as basic as insomnia can create these biochemical imbalances. To disregard malnutrition as a major cause of certain types of depression is to ignore the obvious.

Malnutrition

One cannot discuss the role of therapeutic nutrition in the treatment of depression without discussing malnutrition. In the report "Malnutrition and Hunger in the United States" by the American Medical Association Council on Foods and Nutrition, *malnutrition* is defined as "a state of impaired functional ability or deficient structural integrity or development brought about by a discrepancy between the supply to the body tissues of essential nutrients and calories, and the biologic demand for them."[4]

Relative to other sciences, nutrition is among the youngest, and our present knowledge of human nutritional requirements and the role of nutrition as a therapeutic tool is still limited. The gaps in this knowledge are not being filled as fast as the rate of increase in nutritional and biochemically based disease in the general population.

Malnutrition really exists in two forms, and an individual may suffer from both at the same time. The first form, known as primary malnutrition, is often, though not always, a result of external cultural factors that affect a person's food choices. Factors may include low caloric intake due to food shortages, poverty, poor food selection and meal planning (often resulting from poor nutrition education), contaminated or poisoned foods, and insufficient soil nutrients that result in nutrient-depleted food.

Secondary malnutrition generally results when there is an interference of some type with ingestion, absorption, or utilization of essential nutrients. This is often caused by poor eating habits, crash and yo-yo dieting, and reactions to medications.

A factor that plays a large role in the focus of any treatment for depression is the idea of individual variation; that is, some individuals may require extraordinary levels of specific nutrients that are greatly above what would be required by an average person of similar height or weight. This may also be caused by stress factors that increase nutrient requirements above what would be considered normal levels. This is exactly the problem with individuals with food sensitivity reactions or hypoglycemia. Secondary malnutrition may also result from an excretion of essential nutrients that have not been absorbed properly or destruction in the body of essential nutrients. This may result from eating disorders such as anorexia nervosa and bulimia.

If a person suffers from malnutrition, it is important to determine which form it is, then separate and correct the interrelated factors. Research done at the University of Texas in the 1950s and 1960s by Dr. Roger Williams focused on the concept of human biochemical individuality—the idea that nutrition requirements vary greatly from individual to individual. While one person may do perfectly well on an intake of minimum dietary requirements as established by the scientific community, another person might become ill on the same nutrient-intake levels because he or she requires much higher levels of specific nutritional factors to meet his or her minimum needs. It was Dr. Williams's position that, because of individual nutritional requirements, essentially no one can obtain what he or she needs nutritionally from an average American diet.

Studies have shown that certain groups of diseased individuals on the high end of the spectrum of biochemical need have shown specific deficiencies in certain nutrients. The early studies showed this to be so with alcoholics, drug addicts, and schizophrenics. Recent research indicates this to be so with an ever-greater list of illnesses.

Supplementation

Supplements for the treatment of depression usually fall into three categories: herbal formulas, herbs in combination with vitamins, and combinations of vitamins and substances that occur naturally in the body such as phosphatidylserine (PS), glycerophosphocholine (GPC), citicoline, and acetyl-L-carnitine (ALCAR). The supplements presented in this section generally work by supporting, correcting, or restoring brain function imbalances caused by the factors listed above. These supplements include amino acids, individual vitamins and minerals, or combinations of various supplements such as antioxidants, glandular support formulas, and stress-management formulas. The baffling array of emotional symptoms and the equally baffling array of treatments for the relief of various emotional problems can result in frustration and expense in a search for a "miracle cure" that may not yet exist. In addition, there is often no one treatment that works for everyone. For these reasons, therapies focusing on diet, stress reduction, vitamins, amino acids, and other holistic approaches may require trial and error.

Nutritional products are usually available in a capsule, pill, powder, or liquid form. Though studies are limited, anecdotal evidence indicates that many of the individuals who seem to benefit from prescription serotonin-enhancing medications such as Zoloft, Paxil, and Prozac have responded well to supplementation—particularly vitamin B_6 in doses of 500 milligrams—without side effects. Other helpful nutrients include phosphatidylserine (the major phospholipid found in the brain's cell membranes), L-tryptophan and 5-HTP (both building blocks for serotonin), N-acetyl-serotonin, melatonin, and DL-phenylalanine. Folic acid, vitamin B_{12}, vitamin C, inositol, gingko biloba extract, and acetyl-L-carnitine have been specifically shown to be beneficial in the treatment of depression in the elderly. Supplemental phosphatidylserine may improve depression in the elderly by way of its cortisol-suppressive effect or by improving cell membrane fluidity. Microalgae such as spirulina may also be of great value.

The basic philosophy for using higher-than-average dosages of nutrients to alleviate depression or other mental illness goes back to Dr. Roger Williams's theory that each individual has unique, specific metabolic needs. Some individuals, it is believed, require higher doses of certain nutrients. This is because it is believed that many forms of depression are the result of faulty biochemistry. Thus, the treatment needs to be focused on factors that can correct this imbalance, such as high nutrient doses.

For many individuals, proper dosages of specific nutrients as the answer to depression began with a few pioneering physicians in the 1950s. Treatment based on the concept that faulty biochemistry caused some mental health problems and could be corrected by nutritional means was championed by Linus Pauling, who called this approach orthomolecular medicine.

Pauling defined *orthomolecular medicine* as, "The preservation of good health and the prevention and treatment of disease by varying the concentrations in the human body of the molecules of substances that are normally present, many of them required for life, such as vitamins, essential amino acids, essential fats, and minerals." Dr. Pauling further stated that "a psychiatrist who refuses to try the methods of Orthomeolecular Psychiatry [nutrition as related to mental health], in addition to his usual therapy in the treatment of his patients, is failing in his duty as a physician."[5]

Pauling was no ordinary thinker or researcher. He was the only winner of two unshared Nobel prizes, was cited by Watson and Crick as the codiscoverer of DNA, isolated lysine, and discovered the value of vitamin C as a method of clearing plaque from arteries. Later in his life, Dr. Pauling became a proponent of large doses of vitamin C for a variety of physical and emotional problems. For this, he was attacked by much of the medical establishment. One of his responses was: "Physicians just do what the medical authorities say to do. Of all the professions, the medical profession is the one in which the individual practitioners do the smallest amount of thinking for themselves."[6]

As early as the 1950s and 1960s, Dr. Carl C. Pfieffer and other pioneers in the orthomolecular psychiatry movement discovered that a combination of high-quality whole foods, combined with the correct nutritional supplements, could eliminate most of the mental health problems in the United States. Further research in the 1970s by Dr. John Blass, a physician and biochemist at the Neuropsychiatric Institute at the University of California at Los Angeles, explored this area further.

Most mental health specialists do not support the unguided use of high dosages of specific nutrients as the primary tool for healing depression. There is, however, strong evidence that high doses of certain nutrients may be very helpful for individuals suffering from a specific type of depression—such as that caused by low blood sugar—or an inability to metabolize normal levels of certain nutrients such as magnesium.

Though the use of dietary supplements for therapeutic purposes other than basic nutritional deficiencies has been frowned upon by orthodox medicine, in recent years some of these supplements have been incorporated into conventional and complementary medicine. For example, many pediatricians now recommend folic acid supplements to their patients as a way to reduce the risk of certain birth defects. And ophthalmologists now know that a multivitamin-mineral program that includes zinc can slow the progression of age-related macular degeneration (AMD).

Supplement Absorption

There is a chance that, even if you are on the most effective supplement program possible, you may not receive the benefits of these nutrients. Why? Because, though most gelatin capsules and liquid and powdered supplements are easily digested, many supplement tablets cannot dissolve in your body. These pills pass right through your gastrointestinal tract with little chance of being absorbed by the blood or transported to various tissues whose proper functioning is essential for proper brain function.

According to the *Tufts University Health and Nutrition Newsletter*, "When researchers at the University of Maryland tested nine prescription pre-natal vitamin tablets to see whether the folate they contained would dissolve, only three of them passed muster. Two failed so miserably that they released less than 25 percent of the folate specified on the label."[7] Obviously, a supplement needs to dissolve if it is going to be absorbed.

Dissolvins' standards are set by a nonprofit, independent group of experts in medicine, pharmacy, and related fields known as the U.S. Pharmacopeia (USP). Concerning multivitamin-and-mineral preparations, the USP established that, in order for a pill to "meet the standard" for dissolving, 75 percent of its iron and 75 percent of the vitamin B_2 must dissolve within an hour of being stirred in a weak solution of hydrochloric acid under strict laboratory conditions. Iron and vitamin B_2 were chosen as the standard for the test since they are among the most difficult to dissolve. Thus, if they dissolve, it can be assumed that the other nutrients will dissolve as well. This being the case, what are you to do in order to guarantee the quality and potency of the supplements you are taking? Here are a number of steps:

- Do not pay attention to labels that say SCIENTIFICALLY BLENDED, LABORATORY TESTED, QUALITY AND POTENCY GUARANTEED, or RELEASE ASSURED. All these sayings have virtually no legal meaning.
- When shopping for nutritional supplements, pick the one with the latest expiration date. Nutrients lose their potency over time, and you want to purchase the ones that were manufactured most recently.
- Unless otherwise stated on the label, always take supplements on a full stomach. The food you have eaten will slow the movement

of the nutrients through your gastrointestinal tract, allowing a longer period for them to dissolve and be absorbed.
- Purchase only supplements with USP on the label.

Whatever supplement you use, it is important to maintain the potency and chemical stability of the individual nutrients or herbs. Product storage is thus very important. Do not store them in a bathroom medicine cabinet since the heat and moisture found there may change the action of the supplements. Instead, store them in a cool, dry place, away from direct light, but never freeze them. Needless to say, store them safely out of the reach of children.

Some of the remedies discussed in the remainder of this chapter are folk remedies that have been used successfully for many years. Many are well known throughout published scientific research. If you are presently on medication for emotional or behavioral problems, do not stop taking it on your own.

Remember, genetic differences and biochemical individuality in nutrient absorption and utilization may account for differences in vulnerability to various nutrient deficiencies and differences in individual responses to factors that might contribute to the onset of depression.

Magnesium

Magnesium, along with calcium and iron, is one of the minerals most associated with balancing mood swings. Magnesium is active in the hippocampus (the emotional center of the body) and is essential for the regulation of receptor sites for neurotransmitters. Research has found that magnesium is often low in the blood of people who are seriously, even suicidally, depressed.

Magnesium ions are involved at the very heart of neural synaptic activity. Published reports by the National Institutes of Health (NIH) have stated that depression is an indicator of magnesium deficiency. Early psychological magnesium deficiency symptoms may include confusion, reduced ability to learn, fatigue, apathy, poor memory, anorexia, Tourette syndrome; anxiety (including obsessive-compulsive disorder), irritability, insomnia, grieving, hallucinations, and delirium. Some of these symptoms may occur as part of panic attacks, sometimes with the feeling of imminent death. Early physical magnesium-deficiency symptoms may include muscle twitching, crying, numbness, full-body tingling, and a sustained contraction of the muscles. Even a moderate magnesium deficiency can produce cardiovascular symptoms such as rapid or irregular heartbeat.

The NIH has prepared a list of those foods that are the best sources of magnesium in the U.S. diet. One of the problems with this list is that it does not distinguish between high-magnesium foods and high-magnesium foods that contain even higher levels of calcium. An excess of calcium over magnesium inhibits absorption of magnesium from the diet. Though this might not be a problem for a healthy person on a well-balanced nutritional program, it can create havoc for a depressed individual attempting to create a meal plan full of magnesium-rich foods but who is unaware of the calcium-magnesium factor.

The best food sources of magnesium are peanuts, almonds, kelp and blue-green algae, soy flour, bran flakes, whole wheat, brown rice, avocado, wheat bran, shrimp, tuna, Brazil nuts, cashew nuts, sesame seeds, walnuts, and collard greens.

High stress levels and eating high-fat foods and excessive amounts of calcium can deplete magnesium in your body, leading to depression. One of the key factors to be considered in addressing the magnesium-depression issue is a calcium-magnesium imbalance. Chronic stress with excessive calcium intake and low magnesium intake can cause imbalances in hormones that control calcium levels in the body, thus resulting in depression.

Magnesium Supplementation

Though there is no specific research to support its use over other forms of magnesium, much anecdotal evidence suggests that magnesium glycinate, a nontoxic dietary supplement commonly available in health-food stores and most pharmacies, has been particularly helpful for some depression sufferers. This may be because of its effectiveness in balancing blood sugar problems and maintaining energy related to the controlling of blood sugar.

Magnesium glycinate produces two key benefits. Magnesium, the most prevalent mineral salt inside the cells, plays a key role in the stabilization of the nervous system and in energy production. The amino acid glycine is recognized to have a calming effect on the body. Many people have found that magnesium glycinate has less of a laxative effect than some other magnesium compounds. It is also absorbed more readily than other forms of magnesium. This is probably due to the fact that it is carried into the cells of the body as an amino acid rather than as a mineral, offering the benefits of both magnesium and glycine.

Some individuals I have spoken with have used 200 to 400 milligrams of magnesium glycinate three times daily (once in the morning, once in the early evening, and once at bedtime). When magnesium supplements are taken, the doses are more effective if they are spread out because magnesium is easily lost in the urine.

Glycine, the second component of magnesium glycinate, is a nonessential amino acid but is valuable because it chelates (removes) mercury from the body. Mercury is a toxic metal that can cause many health problems, including emotional instability and especially depression.

If you find that magnesium glycinate does not relieve your depression, explore whether your calcium levels are too high. Excessive calcium intake can reduce magnesium levels and disrupt the entire process. Reduce your calcium intake to the recommended dietary allowance (RDA) and see if this is helpful.

Some depressed people need more calcium because medical laboratory tests show that they are in a negative calcium balance. This is a complex problem for the depressed person. By increasing calcium, they may become more depressed. By decreasing calcium, they may experience health problems related to calcium deficiency.

Magnesium Deficiency

Magnesium deficiency can best be determined through the red blood cell. It is important, when designing a nutritional program for depression, that there is a balance between magnesium and calcium levels. Excessive levels of calcium may prevent magnesium from being fully absorbed into the body. Some individuals are low in magnesium even though their diet seems adequate and they are taking magnesium supplements. Nondietary and nonstress causes of hypomagnesemia (abnormally low levels of magnesium in the body) may result from a deficiency in the mineral boron, and from renal and gastrointestinal disorders that result in malabsorption. If you experience clinical depression and have celiac disease, sprue, radiation injury to the bowel, bowel resection, small bowel bypass, chronic diarrhea, inflammatory bowel disease, endocrine disorder, or neoplasm (an abnormal growth), or if you abuse laxatives or are taking diuretics or drugs such as antibiotics or oral contraceptives, you may be suffering from hypomagnesemia.

Many dietary factors can reduce magnesium absorption or negatively influence magnesium balance. Among these are:

- Excessive doses of vitamin D (perhaps explaining SAD in summer) or calcium supplements may result in renal magnesium loss.
- High intake of cow's milk. This is because the route of absorption in the intestinal tract is the same for these two minerals. If calcium intake is excessive (as is the case with excessive drinking of milk), the calcium will be absorbed in preference to magnesium, and vice versa.
- Excessive consumption of oxalate-rich foods, which can result in the binding of magnesium and preventing it from being absorbed by the body in a usable form. Pekoe tea, spinach, and products made from unhulled sesame seeds are the most commonly ingested oxalate-rich foods.
- Excessive intake of certain nutrients and food items that decrease intestinal absorption of magnesium or increase urinary excretion of this mineral. Among the main culprits are saturated fats, refined sugar, iron, sodium, calcium, alcohol, animal fat, protein, folic acid, caffeine, manganese, phosphorus, potassium, and sodium.
- High intake of the B vitamin riboflavin, which may increase the risk of magnesium deficiency.

People who suffer from lactose intolerance have an added problem. Research indicates that lactose malabsorption from milk products may interfere with the availability of L-tryptophan, thus affecting the body's ability to synthesize serotonin. Both L-tryptophan and serotonin have antidepressant qualities.

Thankfully, depleted magnesium levels can easily be overcome nutritionally. In obese people, magnesium deficiency can become part of a vicious cycle. Overweight and obese people usually eat refined carbohydrates and high-fat foods, which are usually low in magnesium or deplete magnesium in the body. Since magnesium is essential for the metabolizing (burning) of fat, these individuals may experience a magnesium deficiency–based depression while maintaining a diet that increases stress and continued magnesium deficiency, thus leading to greater depression.

Medical literature supports increasing magnesium intake, eating foods rich in the mineral boron, as well as supplementing with both these minerals. These measures will also help prevent the loss of calcium while maintaining magnesium levels.

Magnesium, Sleep, and Depression

Adequate rapid eye movement (REM) sleep is mandatory if a person is to recover from depression. Insomnia is a common symptom associated with depression, and a magnesium deficiency can result from a lack of sleep and can also cause this problem. A key part of this catch-22 is the lowered amounts of growth hormone secretion that occur with sleep deprivation. It has been known for some time that magnesium at bedtime can induce a calm, pleasant sleep. If you suffer from depression and insomnia, take 400 milligrams of magnesium citrate, magnesium malate, or magnesium glycinate at bedtime. It may be of great help.

Many people use melatonin to improve sleep patterns. However, this should be done with caution by anyone who suffers from depression. When a person is sleeping, serotonin is converted to melatonin, and during the waking hours, melatonin is converted to serotonin. The biochemistry of depression prevents certain individuals from being able to effectively convert melatonin into serotonin. In such individuals melatonin levels elevate, aggravating an already existing depression and making the individual extremely drowsy. If using melatonin makes you feel drowsy or increases your depression, either reduce your dosage or cease taking it.

Other Minerals

Deficiencies in a number of minerals can also cause depression. For example, the trace minerals are needed as cofactors for enzymes, and play important roles in turning food into energy, maintaining the electrical balance in bodily fluids, and carrying oxygen in the body. They are part of blood and bone, and allow nerves to transmit messages. The following are the most important minerals and trace minerals for healing depression.

Boron

The mineral boron is important in brain and psychological function, especially through its influence in preserving critical minerals. Boron has been found to be helpful in preventing urinary losses of magnesium and calcium.

When a supplement program included boron, reduced levels of magnesium were needed in order to eliminate depression. In human deficiency studies, boron supplementation improved memory, mental alertness, and mineral metabolism.

The National Academy of Science's Institute of Medicine has set the tolerable upper intake level for boron at 20 milligrams per day. However, no RDA has been established. Good dietary sources of boron include nuts—especially almonds and hazelnuts—and raisins.

People I have spoken with take 6 to 12 milligrams of boron in the morning. Some feel that it has a slightly stimulating, caffeine-like effect and avoid taking it in the evening.

Calcium

After the four main elements—carbon, oxygen, hydrogen, and nitrogen—calcium is probably of greater importance to the human body than any of the alkaline-forming minerals. It plays a key role in building the boney structure of the body, helps the blood to clot, and assists the nervous system, muscular system, and heart in functioning effectively. Calcium is so important in the conversion of chemical energy to muscular contractions and neuromuscular interaction that a deficiency of the mineral can lead to muscle spasms. Calcium is also a neutralizing agent for harmful acids, especially those formed as the result of the consumption of acid-forming foods, including white flour, white sugar, and processed fats.

The best food sources of calcium for a person suffering from depression are buttermilk, yogurt, apricots, and leafy vegetables such as collard greens, cabbage, dandelion, kale, and mustard greens. Certain types of fish, including salmon, are rich in calcium but may also contain mercury, which can aggravate depression in sensitive individuals.

Iron

Iron is an essential constituent of hemoglobin, one of the most important bioelements. The fatigue and listlessness often experienced by persons suffering from depression are often traced to iron deficiency. This is especially true in young women, who often suffer iron loss during menstruation as well as iron deficiency due to an excessive use of iron-deficient processed foods. Loss of appetite and headaches may also be symptoms of iron deficiency. Iron is required for the transportation of oxygen from the lungs to the muscles, brain, and other essential organs.

The best vegetarian food sources of iron include unsulfured molasses, cereals and whole-grain products, sun-dried fruits, dark green leafy vegetables, dry beans, and egg yolks. Consuming lemon juice and taking vitamin-C supplements can help increase the body's ability to absorb iron. Drinking pekoe tea reduces the body's absorption of iron.

Lithium

The use of low-dose lithium salts is a common treatment for depression associated with cyclothymia and other bipolar disorders. Cyclothymia is a mild bipolar disorder that persists over a long period of time. Lithium is a mineral element that is not found in the human diet except in trace amounts (which are related to maintaining an even temperament).

Though lithium has been very helpful to many suffering from bipolar disorder, it should be noted that excess lithium causes hypothyroidism, and hypothyroidism can create a hormonal chain reaction in the body that depletes magnesium levels and ultimately leads to more depression. Some physicians have reduced lithium to lower doses and added high-dose magnesium with positive results. One theory among nutritionally based mental health specialists is that part of the biochemical function of lithium is to increase blood magnesium levels. If this is an accurate theory, then the benefit of lithium in the treatment of bipolar disorder may come not from lithium but from lithium-induced increased magnesium blood levels. This theory might explain why 40 percent of patients with bipolar disorder do not respond to lithium. In these clients, the condition may be caused by a factor other than magnesium deficiency, or their dietary magnesium intake is so low that not even lithium can return it to normal levels.

In recent years, a number of nutritional products have become available that contain lithium carbonate and lithium bromide (derived from the naturally occurring alkali metal) at micronutritional potencies. Though they are at a much lower dosage than pharmaceutically produced lithium salts, these nutritional products may have some value and do not cause the side effects associated with a pharmaceutical dosage of lithium. These products may restore clear, sentient thinking as well as mood stabilization, especially for those individuals who experience potentially explosive and unpredictable mood swings and/or severe bipolar disorder episodes.

Manganese

While excessive intake of manganese can cause a decrease in the absorption of magnesium, deficiency of this metal can affect the proper use of the B-complex vitamins and vitamin C.

Manganese also plays a role in amino acid formation, and a deficiency of the metal can result in depression stemming from low levels of the neurotransmitters serotonin and norepinephrine.

Manganese is also important for those suffering from hypoglycemia since it helps stabilize blood sugar and prevent the mood swings common with the condition.

Potassium

Potassium deficiency is often associated with tearfulness, weakness, fatigue, and depression. Decreased brain levels of potassium have also been found in autopsies of suicides, and a 1981 study discovered that depressed patients were more likely than controls (in studies) to have lowered intracellular potassium. A simple way to increase potassium levels is through the intake of one teaspoon of Morton's Lite Salt every day.

Zinc

Inadequate levels of zinc result in apathy, lack of appetite, and lethargy. When zinc is low, copper in the body can increase to toxic levels, resulting in paranoia and fearfulness. Zinc is also important for healthy pancreatic function and the production of insulin, which is key to controlling hypoglycemia.

Amino Acids

Amino acids are considered the first and most fundamental biofactors of all of life. The human body has about twenty times more amino acids than vitamins and about four times more amino acids than minerals.

One mechanism for reducing or reversing biochemically based depression is to provide certain amino acids through supplementation. These amino acids as well as other dietary precursors can provide and support the body's ability to balance and moderate essential neurotransmitters in the brain and do so without side effects. The following are the most important amino acids for healing depression.

DL-Methionine

A buildup of fat in the liver and arteries can obstruct blood flow to the brain and other essential organs. This reduced blood flow can reduce oxygen leading to the brain and contribute to depression. The essential amino acid DL-methionine (a powerful antioxidant) plays a key role in the breakdown of fats, thus helping to prevent reduced blood flow to the brain. DL-methionine also supports a healthy digestive system and sexual function, and helps to detoxify harmful agents, including lead and other heavy metals, which can contribute to the onset of depression.

DL-Phenylalanine

The amino acid DL-phenylalanine (DLPA) has been found to have excellent antidepressant qualities when compared with various tricyclic antidepressant medications in double-blind studies. It is generally believed that DLPA's effectiveness results from its connection to the elevation of phenylethylamine (PEA) levels in the brain. Increased PEA levels protect the longevity and integrity of endorphins. Endorphins are important neuroproteins involved with pain and mood regulation. Increased PEA levels also affect the balance of L-tyrosine, the amine-neurotransmitter that is the direct precursor of norepinephrine.

5-Hydroxytryptophan

The amino acid 5-hydroxytryptophan (5-HTP) increases brain serotonin concentration. This nutrient is a step closer in the serotonin production pathway, more easily available, and as much as five to ten times more potent than L-tryptophan. It is also more widely available than L-tryptophan, and over 70 percent of 5-HTP is absorbed in the brain.

A number of double-blind studies show that 5-HTP is as effective as antidepressant medication. The generally recommended dose of 5-HTP for adults is 50 to 300 milligrams a day. Children should be started at half this amount. There are seldom any side effects from 5-HTP, but if they do appear, the most common is an upset stomach. To avoid this problem, begin with a low dosage and slowly work your way up. Take 5-HTP on an empty stomach.

L-Theanine

L-theanine is a unique, free-form amino acid that has been found to increase alpha waves, producing mental and physical relaxation. L-theanine is found only in the green tea plant and certain mushrooms. The therapeutic properties associated with L-theanine include its ability to lower stress, diminish symptoms of PMS, decrease anxiety, increase mental acuity, improve learning ability and performance, support the immune system, and increase brain dopamine levels.

Based on the results of clinical studies, some holistic physicians recommended taking L-theanine in single dosages in the range of 50 to 200 milligrams. It is suggested that subjects with higher levels of anxiety take a dose at the higher end of the effective range (100 to 200 milligrams).

L-Tryptophan

L-tryptophan is found in milk products, meat, and eggs. Nutritionally based mental health specialists have favored it in dosages of 1,000 to 3,000 milligrams daily because it has helped their patients decrease aggressive behavior, improve mood, and sleep better—all without side effects. One might ask, "If tryptophan is so abundant in food, why bother taking it in supplement form?" A primary reason is that only a small amount—3 percent of dietary L-tryptophan—ever enters the brain. Instead, the body uses it to make vitamin B_3 and proteins. Thus, food does not supply a dosage high enough to obtain the therapeutic effects required for someone suffering from clinical depression.

It is important to note that L-tryptophan has a controversial history that is unwarranted. It was removed from the marketplace a number of years ago owing to a number of deaths from eosinophilia-myalgia syndrome (EMS), a rare blood disease caused by one contaminated batch from a single manufacturer, the Showa Denka Corporation in Japan. The Centers for Disease Control and the Mayo Clinic cleared the role of L-tryptophan in the EMS outbreak in 1992. In fact, L-tryptophan is still safely being used in infant formulas and parenteral intravenous (IV) solutions, all of which are approved by the FDA. L-tryptophan has been reapproved by the FDA by prescription.

Many nutritionists recommend using 5-HTP because it is a direct precursor to serotonin (5-hydroxy-tryptamine, or 5-HT) and considered to be as much as ten times more powerful in producing serotonin than L-tryptophan. Vitamin B_6 serves as a cofactor for the conversion of 5-HTP to 5-HT, which is why many nutritional supplements formulated for the treatment of depression contain vitamin B_6.

L-Tyrosine

L-tyrosine is a naturally occurring amino acid that is a key factor in the formation of important neurotransmitters, especially dopamine. Dopamine is an important factor for the "concentration and thinking" functions of the prefrontal cortex of the brain. Studies have demonstrated that consuming L-tyrosine enhances the production of dopamine, norepinephrine, and epinephrine, and may alleviate certain symptoms of depression, as well as improve alertness and focus. Studies performed by the U.S. military have shown that consuming an L-tyrosine supplement may also enhance cognitive performance.

L-tyrosine accounts for as much as 90 percent of the production of these neurotransmitters, which are synthesized directly from L-tyrosine. Some nutritional physicians prescribe 500 to 1,500 milligrams of L-tyrosine two to three times a day for depressed adults, and 100 to 500 milligrams two to three times a day for depressed children under the age of ten.

Some researchers believe that the use of certain nutrients and herbs— such as L-tyrosine and the herb St. John's wort—can enhance the half-life of certain neurotransmitters, naturally relieving the effect of daily symptoms of mental and physical burnout that can lead to depression. However, there are no definitive studies indicating what the most effective dosage of L-tyrosine might be. Many nutritionists believe that consuming 2 to 3 grams of L-tyrosine with a high-complex-carbohydrate meal can help prevent the sluggish feeling and decreased alertness that is sometimes caused by increased levels of serotonin.

No known side effects have been reported with L-tyrosine and, thus far, it has been shown to be extremely safe and effective.

S-Adenosyl-Methionine

S-adenosyl-methionine, more commonly known as SAM-e, is one of the most effective natural antidepressants. It is better tolerated and works faster than many tricylic antidepressant drugs. Its effectiveness comes from its ability to enhance the functioning of monoamines such as dopamine, serotonin, and gamma-aminobutyric acid (GABA). In a healthy person with balanced brain chemistry, adequate amounts of SAM-e are produced from the amino acid methionine. In depressed individuals, however, this synthesis seems to be impaired. Numerous double-blind, placebo-controlled studies have found that, when taken as a supplement, SAM-e enhances dopamine and serotonin function and promotes clinical improvement in depressed patients with fewer side effects than antidepressant drugs.

The usual dosage of SAM-e begins at 200 milligrams two times per day, for several days, and is gradually increased to a dose of 400 milligrams four times per day. The nutrient can cause nausea and vomiting. If this happens, reduce the dosage. SAM-e supplementation may increase manic symptoms and thus should not be taken by patients with bipolar disorder.

Other Nutrients

Though the vitamins, minerals, and amino acids discussed thus far may have a major influence on relieving depression, there are many nutrients that, though not essential, can play a subtle role in the biochemistry of the disorder. Other nutrients serve as precursors for the formation of even more nutrients that can relieve depression. The nutrients mentioned here only scratch the surface, yet they are important to note.

Inositol

Inositol supports many different body functions, particularly nerve, muscle, and brain function. It works closely with other nutrients, especially choline, vitamins B_6 and B_{12}, betaine (trimethylglycine), folacin, and methionine. Inositol is present in all animal tissues, with the highest levels in the heart and brain. The cerebrospinal fluid, spinal cord nerves, and brain contain large amounts of inositol. Various studies indicate that depressed individuals generally have much-lower-than-normal levels of inositol in their spinal fluid. Initial evidence indicates that inositol might be helpful in the treatment of depression.

Food sources of inositol include whole grains, beans, nuts, seeds, cantaloupe, and citrus fruits (with the exception of lemon). I recommend these foods as dietary sources for inositol. Also, foods rich in a substance called phytic acid are a good source of inositol since phytic acid, when acted on by bacteria in the digestive tract, releases inositol.

Some nutritionally based physicians have reported that inositol has a sedating quality that solves many insomnia and anxiety problems, especially in those suffering from hypoglycemia. Some individuals may suffer from stress-induced depression and may have stress-elevated blood pressure.

Inositol may be helpful in bringing this hypertension back to normal. Some individuals with depression have high copper and low zinc levels. Supplementation with pure inositol (not the phosphate ester of inositol) favors absorption of zinc.

In depression and panic disorder, the recommended dosage of inositol is 12 grams daily. A well-balanced whole food diet of 2,500 calories would contain 1,000 milligrams of inositol. Dosages of up to 18 grams daily have been tried in various experiments for various conditions with no serious ill-effects being reported. I am not suggesting taking a dosage of this level. Do not take this high a dosage without the guidance of a physician.

Sadly, many individuals who are depressed, especially those who are in recovery from excessive alcohol use, are heavy drinkers of coffee, tea, cocoa, and other caffeine-containing substances. Unfortunately, caffeine intake in large quantities may create an inositol shortage, which itself can contribute to depression.

According to the book *Vitamins, Herbs, Minerals, and Supplements* by H. Winter Griffith, M.D. (Perseus, 2000), inositol is best taken as inositol monophosphate capsules with meals or one to one and a half hours after meals unless otherwise directed by your doctor.

Caution: No long-term safety studies have been performed on inositol. Consult your physician if you have tingling, numbness, alternating feelings of cold and hot in feet and hands, and/or diabetes with peripheral neuropathy pain.

Nicotinamide Adenine Dinucleotide

Nicotinamide adenine dinucleotide (NADH) is a compound produced by the body that stimulates the brain's production of dopamine and norepinephrine. In one study, NADH was found to alleviate depression. A potent antioxidant NADH is also involved in cellular energy production.

Phenylethylamine

Phenylethylamine (PEA) is an endogenous neuroamine that is normally found in the human brain and has been found to have mood-elevating effects, including the reduction of depression. Research indicates that some depressed patients have decreased urinary levels of PEA. This suggests a deficiency in this factor. PEA, which has amphetamine-like properties, is metabolized from the amino acid D-phenylalanine, which does not normally occur in the body or in food. A large proportion of this amino acid is also converted to the amino acid L-tyrosine. Studies indicate that the amino acid phenylalanine not only reduces depression through the production of PEA but, with the amino acid tyrosine, builds dopamine and norepinephrine levels. These are important neurotransmitters in the brain.

A study published in the *Journal of Neuropsychiatry and Clinical Neuroscience* found that PEA was shown to relieve depression in 60 percent of depressed patients.[8] Some researchers believe that a PEA deficiency may be a cause of a common form of depressive illness. Patients in the study who suffered from major depressive episodes and received PEA treatment responded to a PEA intake of 10 to 60 milligrams orally per day. It should be noted that the patients also received 10 milligrams of selegiline per day to prevent rapid PEA destruction. It was found that, in most patients, the antidepressant response had been maintained and the effective dosage did not change with time. PEA not only improved the mood of the patients as rapidly as amphetamine, but also did not produce the tolerance associated with that drug that often results in an increase in dosage. PEA produced sustained relief of depression in most of the patients, even some that had been unresponsive to standard treatments for depression. And there were no apparent side effects.

Research on exercise and depression indicates that running and jogging increases PEA levels as well.

Phosphatidylserine

Phosphatidylserine (PS) is a natural substance that can influence depression in the elderly. It is a phospholipid derived from lecithin that is an essential component of the cell membrane. The brain can manufacture PS, which plays an important role in maintaining the fluidity and integrity of brain cell membranes. PS allows nutrients and oxygen to enter the brain more easily and also stimulates release of acetylcholine and dopamine. However, if there is an essential fatty acid, folic acid, or vitamin B_{12} deficiency, the brain may be unable to manufacture enough of it.

Some physicians recommend dosages of 100 milligrams twice a day for two weeks. Then, if needed, 100 milligrams three times a day for memory.

Phosphatidylcholine

Phosphatidylcholine (PC), also known as lecithin, is the major fat in the cell membranes. An emulsifier, it is believed to help keep the bloodstream clear of fatty deposits. PC is high in linoleic acid, which is necessary for normal growth and health. It also supplies the body with choline, which is essential for the proper functioning of the liver and the brain. In addition, it increases the levels of the neurotransmitter acetylcholine. Supplementation with PC therefore may help in the treatment of some manic conditions.

Phosphatidylcholine is produced in the body. Good food sources of the nutrient include egg yolks, liver, and soybeans.

Pregnenolone

Pregnenolone, as 3-alpha-hydroxyl-5-beta-pregnen-20-one is more popularly known, is an obscure, natural hormone, made primarily in the adrenal glands but also in the ovaries, skin, liver, brain, and testicles. Preg, among other things, has been shown to improve energy levels, memory, and mood. Research indicates that pregnenolone can partially reduce the need for antidepressants. In his book *Pregnenolone: Nature's Feel Good Hormone* (Avery, 1997), Ray Sahelian, M.D., addresses the possibility that pregnenolone might be of value in treating depression in the elderly. He says, in part, "These antidepressents may often help, but they will not address the primary problem if the low mood is a result of a deficiency of brain steroid hormones. I believe that preg will eventually be found to have a role in treating depression and will be used by itself, or in combination with hormones, vitamins and nutrients."[9]

Anecdotal evidence indicates that as little as 10 milligrams of preg can create a stable, constant mood. Much of the research on preg is in the early stages, but it is certainly a source of healing depression that needs to be explored.

Allergies and Depression

Food additives can cause allergic and sensitivity reactions that disrupt the subtle balance in normal brain chemistry while creating a host of physical reactions that can cause physical stress, emotional confusion, and depression. Foods can cause these reactions, too.

According to *Taber's Encyclopedic Medical Dictionary*, an allergy is an abnormal response of body tissues to a specific protein (allergen), which in a nonreactive person will, in about the same amount, create no response.

The word *allergy* means "altered reaction," and there are two prevailing views concerning what the biochemical application of the definition of *allergy* should be. The mainstream or *reductionist* school of thought insists that, for a reaction to be allergic, there must be a demonstrable immunological mechanism underlying the altered reaction—for example, antibodies forming in opposition to the allergen or antigen. The other school of thought—and the one embraced by a good part of the alternative and complementary medical community—believes that it is enough simply to recognize a specific substance as the source of an individual's reaction.

Whichever definition one wishes to use, the experience is the same. Reactions such as swelling, itching, depression, mood swings, or other mental responses result because the body identifies this food or substance as an invader or as a potentially dangerous substance, and then reacts to the intrusion.

How Hypersensitivity Reactions and Allergies Can Lead to Depression

In addition to the six essential nutrients and many other nonessential nutrients that are found in food, many commercially manufactured foods contain synthetic chemical compounds, otherwise known as *additives*, that have been put into the foods during processing. The problem with synthetic, nonnutritional additives is that they can cause depression, mood swings, and other emotional problems in certain individuals who are extremely sensitive to these chemicals in food and who will react to them. Among the psychological and emotional symptoms that can be tied to allergic or sensitivity responses are depression, sadness or despondency, anxiety, phobias, irritability, loneliness, hopelessness, worry, shyness, and brooding. Mental conditions are confusion, mental fatigue, stress, and attention deficit. Physical symptoms include headaches, heart pain and palpitations, hyperactivity, and physical fatigue.

Delayed Allergy

Delayed allergy results when something that has been eaten or inhaled consistently over a period of time is suddenly reacted to where there was no previous reaction. To isolate this type of condition, you should keep a detailed diary of your meals. This diary should include which foods you eat; when you eat each food item; how much you eat of each item; and your reactions, if any, to each food, even if the reaction is seemingly insignificant. This way you can better isolate specific symptoms, associate the reactions with certain foods, and then avoid those foods.

Although this method for identifying food sensitivity is obviously inexpensive, it is not as accurate as the more formal laboratory tests used today. You can confirm an allergen by abstaining from any foods that you believe might be causing the reaction.

When the symptoms subside, avoid that chemical or food for about a week. Then add a dose of the avoided food or drink and observe the results. If the same emotional or physical symptoms occur within thirty minutes, you have identified the culprit.

Avoidance of the allergen is recommended. This system can be applied to a whole range of chemicals, as well as beverages and foods. It is an objective, repeatable approach. It is also a reflection of Dr. Roger Williams's theory of biochemical individuality. Williams stated that different foods may produce different symptoms in the same person, and the same food will produce differing symptoms in different individuals.

Another inexpensive, self-testing method is the pulse test. Dr. Arthur Coca, an immunologist, developed this test when he discovered that there is a rapid increase in the heartbeat—twenty or more beats above normal—when people eat foods they're sensitive to. To take the test, take your resting pulse rate when you awake in the morning. Do this by taking a watch with a second hand and count the number of beats in a sixty-second period. (A normal pulse reading is fifty to seventy beats per minute.) Next, eat a food you suspect is causing your allergy and take another pulse reading. Finally, take your pulse again after fifteen minutes. If your pulse rate has increased more than ten beats per minute, you are probably sensitive or allergic to the food. Again, eliminate the suspect food from your diet for at least two weeks. If you are allergic or sensitive to this food, your symptoms should subside.

Initially, you may not even notice a connection between a food you eat and the physical or emotional symptoms you may experience. You might eat a certain food and three or four days later begin to experience fatigue, depression, headaches, or other symptoms. Many nutritionists and physicians report that people who constantly eat the same foods on a regular basis over an extended period of time can develop a sensitivity or allergy to those foods. Food sensitivity may also develop from weak adrenal gland function, low digestive enzymes, and poor nutrient absorption.

Allergy Testing

Three laboratory tests that are commonly used today are the radioallergosorbent test, cytotoxic food testing, and provocation-neutralization. The radioallergosorbent test, simply known as RAST, is an inhalant test that determines antibody levels for specific allergens that might be present in your bloodstream. RAST not only identifies which inhalants cause allergic responses, but also shows the degree of severity of each response. Therefore, it is especially helpful in identifying the appropriate treatment.

In cytotoxic food testing, a doctor or technician uses a blood sample to test the reaction of your blood cells to 150 or more different foods. Using a microscope, the doctor or technician determines your allergy to foods by observing how severely each food destroys white blood cells. Cytotoxic tests seem to be less specific than the results of RAST testing.

Provocation-neutralization is generally administered by a physician who specializes in the treatment of multiple chemical sensitivities. Various concentrations of suspected substances are placed under the tongue or injected into the skin of the patient. After this procedure, if the patient reports any symptoms, the test is then considered positive. The next step is to give the patient various concentrations of different substances, which may include chemicals, food extracts, hormones, and other natural substances until a dose is found that eliminates or "neutralizes" the symptoms. A combination of substances may be prescribed as "neutralizing" agents. The "neutralization" approach is similar in some ways to the desensitization process used by mainstream allergists. The diagnosis of sensitivities is less scientific with multiple chemical sensitivities since greater respect is given to the subjective judgments of the physician.

Do not ignore allergies and sensitivities as a cause of your depression. The evaluation tools described above will help define whether this is an area requiring special attention.

Keep in Mind

You require over forty different nutrients. These include amino acids (from proteins), essential fatty acids (from fats and oils), and sources of energy (calories from carbohydrates, fats, and proteins). Of course, water, vitamins, and minerals are also essential. Don't be afraid to experiment with amounts of this or that until you see what combination of nutrients works best for you. Also, it may be helpful to seek individual consultation to learn more about the most effective regime for your special nutritional needs. Recognize, too, that your nutritional requirements will vary at different times in your life—and at different seasons of the year—and that they are greatly affected by the stress of any significant changes in your life.

Be Responsible

Self-care is important, but there is an old saying that the doctor who treats himself has a fool for a patient. What I said about choosing herbs in Chapter 3 applies to nutritional supplements as well. If you are depressed and are considering using a nutritional approach to treat your depression, talk with a mental health care professional with a knowledge of depression as well as nutrition. This is especially so if you are suicidal or chronically depressed.

Though there are many specific nutritional and herbal factors that have been shown to reduce depression, it is unwise to base your program simply on a hodge-podge of supplements. Whether using amino acids, magnesium, or St. John's wort to treat depression, the underlying cause is not being addressed. Any factor in depression that is not addressed at the source will require higher supplementation doses in order to bring about an effect. Unbalanced megadoses of certain nutrients have potential risks as well.

Though many nutrients can be taken in large doses without any significant side effects, long-term studies are still not yet available on them and they may, in fact, be shown to have some side effects. This is the argument that some physicians use to limit or restrict the use of nutritional therapies. Unfortunately, these same physicians are often completely ignorant of the benefits that a well-balanced nutritional program can bring about for a person suffering from depression. I am not suggesting that you avoid nutritional therapies and replace them with antidepressant drugs. I am only pointing out that the key to healing depression is to explore the causative factors that can lead to depression and address them as fully as possible before deciding on a supplement program.

Do not use any nutritional approach as a replacement for competent medical care. This is important for your safety and for the development of an integrated and comprehensive treatment plan. If you are using supplements, become informed about the products, their ingredients, and what is known scientifically about them. Never hesitate to request information from the product manufacturer or distributor.

Isolating Nutritional Deficiencies

There are hundreds of symptoms that can be directly traced to nutritional deficiencies. Everything from brittle nails, loss of the sense of smell, hair loss, poor digestion, and depression may be caused by the lack of a single nutrient. Nutrient deficiencies can be discovered by medical testing of blood, urine, hair, and through energetic-vibrational based approaches including kinesiological muscle testing (see Chapter 9).

Once a deficiency has been isolated, it must be determined if this condition is a result of poor food choices or of other factors, which may include poor digestion and nutrient absorption. Based on the defined cause, treatment will usually involve dietary modification or supplementation of the involved nutrient. Digestive evaluation and specific nutritional protocols will also generally be required to correct this situation.

An effective nutrition program to reduce depression should focus on foods that are rich in vegetable proteins and complex carbohydrates such as whole grains, beans, and raw nuts and seeds. Choose vegetables, fruits, and unrefined cereals and flours whenever possible. This will reduce mood swings by providing your brain with a steady supply of glucose. For additional guidelines, see "Nutritional Tips to Reduce Depression" below.

Nutritional Tips to Reduce Depression

- Avoid drinking alcohol of any kind. It can create an imbalance in the pancreas, upsetting blood sugar levels and exaggerating an already existing state of depression.
- To increase omega-3 and essential fatty acid levels, add flaxseeds (or blue-green algae) to your salads, breakfast cereals, and protein shakes.
- Increase your intake of essential nutrients and fiber by eating lots of green leafy vegetables.
- Avoid food that is high on the glycemic index. These foods can create an imbalance in the pancreas, upsetting blood sugar levels and aggravating an already existing state of depression.
- Eat sea vegetables to obtain small levels of absorbable lithium, to increase your mineral intake and balance your thyroid gland.
- Avoid white, brown, and turbinado sugar; maple syrup; and other types of refined or concentrated sugar.
- Eat one bar of low-sugar, or maltitol-sweetened dark chocolate daily. Chocolate is a great source of phenylalanine, a building block of some neurotransmitters.
- Take a soy-, wheat-, and dairy-free multivitamin-and-mineral supplement.
- Eat five to six small meals throughout the day rather than three large meals. This will help stabilize blood sugar and pancreatic function.
- Avoid fast foods, junk foods, all other highly processed foods, and foods high in fat and refined carbohydrates. Many of these foods contain artificial ingredients that can cause food sensitivity reactions.
- Reduce your use of vegetable oils (with the exception of high-EFA oils such as flaxseed and walnut oils, and monounsaturates such as olive oil).

- Use antioxidant supplementation to reduce free radical formation.
- Avoid artificial colors, flavors, and preservatives in your food. Certain chemicals are excitotoxins, specifically affecting the brain in a way that makes them especially problematic. Two of the most common culprits are the noncaloric sweetener aspartame and the flavor-enhancer monosodium glutamate (MSG). MSG is commonly added to Chinese food.

My friend Jerrold Mundis, whom I quoted in Chapter 1, told me about his own program for depression. He says:

My own personal regimen for depression, with details, is:

1. SAM-e, 400 milligrams a day, upped to 500 to 600 milligrams a day in the winter.
2. A light box used to reduce SAD and bring full-spectrum light to the brain and body at those times of the year when natural sunlight is in short supply. I begin in mid-September with fifteen minutes a day of 10,000 lux (a measurement of the intensity of the light) escalating to a full two hours a day by winter solstice and backing down to fifteen minutes a day, ending in mid-March.
3. Working cognitive techniques as needed.

I also find that being careful to keep a normal daytime schedule rather than a night schedule (which my biorhythms have always preferred) has a positive prophylactic effect.[10]

As you can see, treating depression nutritionally involves much more than just taking some vitamins, but if integrated holistically into a treatment program, nutrition is invaluable in the healing of chronic depression.

5  DEPRESSION, IMMUNITY, AND THE GLANDULAR SYSTEM

From the moment your development begins in the womb to the last second of your life, there is a constant interaction between your hormones, your immune system, and your brain. Our hormonal levels are always in a state of flux. With or without stress, every moment there are biochemical reactions in our brain affecting our brain chemistry and, as a result, our moods. As we experience stress at one level or another, our muscles tense up or relax, hormone levels rise and drop in different concentrations, and blood sugar levels increase or decrease. Without these complex checks and balances within our bodies, our moods would be completely erratic or unable to shift as situations require.

Immunity is greatly influenced by the glandular system, especially through the hypothalamus and the thyroid gland. Since the immune system, the central nervous system, and the glandular system play such important roles in emotional health, it is important to explore the association among these systems as they relate to depression.

Hypoglycemia

It is generally recognized that what you eat and when and how you eat it can influence how your brain produces serotonin, dopamine, and nor-epinephrine—the neurotransmitters—which, in turn, affect your behavior and mental attitude. Thus there is no one perfect diet for maximum brain and emotional function.

Some individuals—owing to specific glandular imbalances—have a difficulty or inability to stabilize blood sugar levels, resulting in hyper-

and hypoglycemia. Many individuals with low blood sugar may experience many emotional problems.

Studies have shown that even the healthiest person will experience mood shifts based on how he or she combines different foods. Much of this happens through how the pancreas and the adrenal glands respond to stress or nutrient deficiencies. Through conscious eating and proper food combining, you can control your moods and emotional responses instead of having them control you.

One of the most common glandular factors in depression is a condition called *hypoglycemia,* or low blood sugar. Symptoms of hypoglycemia are episodic and are directly related to the time and content of the last meal. Psychological symptoms of hypoglycemia include absentmindedness, loss of memory and/or concentration, moodiness, insomnia, nightmares, anxiety, depression, paranoia, fears, restlessness, irritability, indecisiveness, and confusion. The symptoms associated with hypoglycemia are sometimes mistaken for symptoms caused by conditions not related to blood sugar. For example, unusual stress and anxiety can cause excess production of catecholamines (dopamine and norepinephrine), resulting in symptoms similar to those caused by hypoglycemia, but having no relation to blood sugar levels.

There are many causes for hypoglycemia besides nutritional factors. However, nutrition can play an important role in reducing emotional symptoms caused by hypoglycemia. This is especially so when the source for the symptoms is adrenocortical insufficiency—especially adrenocortical insufficiency aggravated by stress. Adrenocortical insufficiency can influence the relationship between the pancreas, insulin production, and how foods are metabolized. This will define how easily glucose enters the circulation and is brought to the brain.

You can determine whether or not you have hypoglycemia by taking a glucose tolerance test from a holistic physician. If you are diagnosed with this condition, you can stabilize your emotions and mood swings by using foods low on what is called the glycemic index, in combination with herbs that stabilize the pancreas and adrenal glands. One of my favorite herb formulas includes equal parts of blueberry leaf, licorice root, juniper berry, and ginger root.

The Glycemic Index

The glycemic index is a scale for measuring the effect an individual food has on blood sugar (glucose) levels. The index has been utilized for years by diabetics and hypoglycemics as a way to predict how their bodies will respond to certain foods. With this approach, it is easier to control sugar-based mood swings and emotional changes as you organize a healthy meal plan.

Functional hypoglycemia is a debilitating metabolic disorder resulting from an abnormally low level of glucose in the blood. Since the brain cell's only source of fuel is glucose, abnormally low blood glucose levels can create a state of decreased energy, fatigue, and sugar starvation in the brain and nervous system. This sugar starvation is a major cause of clinical depression. Luckily, this condition can be totally controlled by a specially structured diet combined with nutritional and herbal therapy.

Although hypoglycemia is not the cause of all or even most depressions, almost every symptom that is associated with clinical depression is a symptom that is known to result, in some individuals, because of low blood sugar.

So much of how our body and mind functions is affected by blood sugar levels that it is surprising that more mental health professionals do not investigate it or know much about it.

Glucose is the simplest form of sugar and is formed when other more complex sugars and carbohydrates are digested. For instance, there is lactose (milk sugar), fructose (fruit sugar, and in its most refined and concentrated form, high-fructose corn syrup), and sucrose (refined from cane or beet sugar). These sugars are digested and broken down into the simple sugar found in the blood called glucose.

Levels of glucose in the blood are maintained by the body through the balancing of two opposing factors—insulin and insulin antagonists. When we eat any food containing sugar or starch, our digestive system breaks nutrients down, and as they are absorbed into the bloodstream, blood sugar begins to rise.

In a healthy individual, the pancreas releases insulin, a hormone that removes the blood sugar and carries it to the liver, where it is stored as a form of liver starch called glycogen. This is where insulin antagonists enter the picture. These substances, which include glucocorticoids, adrenalin, the hormone glucagon, and various growth hormones, are produced by the body and serve many functions, including the raising of blood sugar. Glucagon, for instance, will stimulate the conversion of glycogen to glucose in the liver and pass it back into the bloodstream, where it will be carried throughout the body as a fuel source for the cells. In this way, the body has the fuel it needs and blood sugar levels never rise too high or sink too low.

It is still not clear what specific malfunction in the glucose tolerance process brings about hypoglycemia. Some researchers believe it is probably the result of a number of malfunctions. Whatever the cause, the result is an inability of the body to maintain a balance between insulin and its antagonists. According to most current research, there are five major causes of functional hypoglycemia:

1. Stress
2. The excessive use of stimulants (caffeine, tobacco)
3. Certain pharmaceutical agents
4. Refined carbohydrates (white and brown sugar, white rice, and the refined flour products often found in bread and pasta products)
5. Deficiencies in key nutrients that are essential for carbohydrate metabolism and specifically the proper functioning of insulin

Key Nutrients for Preventing and Treating Hypoglycemia-Based Depression

In Chapter 4, we discussed various nutrients that might influence depression. In addition to magnesium, inositol, and various amino acids, the mineral chromium and various enzymes also have a great influence on mental health. In fact over 50,000 enzymes in the human body require the presence of specific metallic trace elements in order to function. Many of these are frequently overlooked by physicians.

Original research done by Dr. Henry Schroeder showed that low levels of the mineral chromium resulted in an increase in blood sugar levels. Research done in the late 1970s and early 1980s by Dr. William Mertz, chairman of the Nutrition Institute of the U.S. Department of Agriculture (USDA), proved that chromium was essential for the body to utilize sugar. When chromium was deficient, insulin was unable to allow sugar to pass into the cells for use as an energy source. In the early 1970s, further research discovered what came to be known as glucose tolerance factor (GTF). GTF, which contains three amino acids, nicotinic acid, and chromium, is required for insulin to function properly and may be key to effective carbohydrate metabolism, without which hypoglycemia or diabetes develops.

One of the most effective ways to get chromium is through the mineral complex chromium picolinate. This is a component of glucose tolerance factor, which supports insulin in regulating blood sugar levels more efficiently. A diet that is high in refined sugar and other carbohydrates and low in chromium will eventually lead to a deficiency in the mineral and can lead to blood sugar metabolism disorders such as diabetes or hypoglycemia. In the case of the latter condition, clinical depression may result.

Herbs for Hypoglycemia

Gymnema sylvestre is a popular herb in India that has been used for thousands of years for various blood sugar metabolism disorders. It is believed that the herb works by dulling the ability of the taste buds to recognize sweets, causing a reduction in sweet cravings. Gymnema also helps stabilize insulin production, helping to reduce many of the symptoms associated with this condition. One study showed that gymnema restimulated the beta cells in the pancreas to produce insulin in insulin-dependent diabetics.

There are a variety of Chinese herbal formulas that are effective in the treatment of depression. Some Chinese herbs do this by somehow reducing blood sugar levels. Tremella (*Tremella fuciformis*), a mushroom also called "silver ear" or "white jerry leaf," is popular in China for many health problems. However, recent research indicates that the fungus helps lower blood glucose by improving the secretion of insulin.

When dealing with chronic depression, these herbs should be treated with the same seriousness as a physician's antidepressant prescription, since the specific formula and dosage of these herbs need to be consistently monitored by a trained professional.

Diagnosing Hypoglycemia

How can a person know if his or her depression is caused by low blood sugar as opposed to some other factor? This is not easy to accomplish; however, there are certain indicators to look out for. Though the symptoms will vary from individual to individual, those suffering from reactive hypoglycemia will virtually always experience chronic physical and mental fatigue. Hypoglycemia, at one time or another, has been connected to almost every symptom that one might suffer in chronic depression including anxiety, insomnia, sexual dysfunction, mood swings, irritability, and depression, especially for those between the ages of thirty and forty. When a person experiences these symptoms in an episodic pattern—especially in relation to the content and time of their last meal—and no mental or physical abnormality can be isolated, hypoglycemia must be explored as the cause. This is especially so if there is some family history of mental illness, obesity, alcoholism, or diabetes.

Since blood glucose is the fuel used by the body's cells, a condition of low cell fuel resulting from an abnormal metabolism of glucose results in numerous psychological and physical symptoms including depression. Most healthy people will experience mood changes as a result of a nutritionally deficient diet or from hunger. But with a simple change to a well-balanced diet, blood sugar is stabilized and mood becomes stabilized as well. This is not the case when a person suffers from hypoglycemia. With this condition, the lowered blood sugar is continuous or chronic, as are the symptoms related to this condition, which often include depression.

The development of the glucose tolerance test enabled physicians to specifically define whether or not a person was subject to low blood sugar. The patient drinks a measured amount of glucose, generally served in a sweet drink. Several blood samples are then drawn over a five- to six-hour period. The purpose of this is to determine both the normal blood sugar level of the individual, as well as the ability of the body to return to and maintain this blood sugar level or a level close to normal over a six-hour period.

Some physicians who were skeptical to begin with criticized this approach to diagnosing hypoglycemia. They pointed out that some individuals may exhibit symptoms of hypoglycemia and yet show blood sugar levels just a little below normal. Other individuals may have exhibited no or few symptoms at all and yet showed a greater drop in blood sugar than might have been expected. Harvey M. Ross, M.D., addresses this very issue in his classic book *Fighting Depression*:

> In making the diagnosis of hypoglycemia, too often the results are scrutinized for one level that falls below some predetermined point which has been designated as normal. In my experience using this criterion, over 90 percent of treatable hypoglycemia will be missed. And it seems that, the more hypoglycemia is considered a fad, the lower the

blood sugar must fall in the estimation of some physicians before they
will make a diagnosis of hypoglycemia.[1]

With this difficulty in creating a specific point in which blood sugar
levels would be considered normal, a new approach to interpreting the
glucose tolerance test had to be developed. Actually, Dr. Roger Williams
had already addressed this issue in other areas of health when he developed the concept of human biochemical individuality. When applied to
the glucose tolerance test, the idea that a varying range of "normal blood
sugar levels" might exist from individual to individual made sense. While
one person may show no symptoms with one response to the test, another person might become ill on this same level because they responded
differently on the test.

So the dilemma still remained. Even if the glucose tolerance test was
an effective tool for diagnosing hypoglycemia, how would a physician define what might be the "normal blood sugar level" for that individual? The
answer came from Dr. H. Salter, who called a situation of this type "relative hypoglycemia." He hypothesized that, if an individual refrained from
eating or drinking at least twelve hours prior to the test and then gave a
blood sample, this "fasting" blood sugar level would be the "normal level"
for that person. With this standard in place, other criteria could achieve
greater meaning for the physician conducting the test. According to Dr.
Salter, once the fasting level was established, if the blood sugar level fell
more than 20 milligrams below the fasting level and the patient experienced any hypoglycemic symptoms, the client could be diagnosed as suffering from relative hypoglycemia. Dr. Salter also noted that if the client
experienced hypoglycemic symptoms at the same time that blood sugar
levels were to drop 50 milligrams percent or more in any one hour, that
this person should be considered to have relative hypoglycemia as well.

Dr. Ross also notes that there are additional criteria that might indicate relative hypoglycemia, including the failure of the blood sugar to elevate 50 percent (not 50 milligrams percent) above the fasting blood
sugar level (this appears as a flat curve on the test results); and if there is
a rapid elevation in blood sugar after the second hour. (This would appear as a sawtooth curve on the test results.) Proper evaluation of low
blood sugar will require that the physician monitor the body's levels of
blood sugar, insulin, and cortisol over a three-hour period after consuming a high-carbohydrate meal.

Glucose tolerance testing is not an exact science but it is an extremely valuable tool. Since depression is one of the most common symptoms experienced by hypoglycemic patients, any person who experiences depression without a clear cause should consider exploring low blood sugar. For the person who is chronically depressed and has found no resolution to his struggle, the discovery that hypoglycemia is the culprit may open the door to emotional freedom.

Correcting Malfunctions of Blood Sugar Metabolism

As was mentioned earlier, glucose is the key fuel for the cells, and glucose is rapidly produced from refined carbohydrates, especially sugar. If there were some way to bring glucose into the body at a slower rate, it would require less insulin and thus produce less of a shock to the glucose tolerance mechanisms.

The dietary program that seems to get this result and thus the best response from those suffering from hypoglycemia-based depression is a high protein–low carbohydrate, whole-food lactovegetarian diet. This is a modified form of the original diet designed by Dr. Seale Harris in the 1920s.

On this diet the body gets most of its glucose not from carbohydrates but from proteins and fats. These moderate, whole-food, carbohydrate-balanced meals help the hypoglycemic reduce depression and other associated symptoms by preventing the extreme rise in blood sugar after eating, something that often happens with high-carbohydrate diets.

A healthy person with normal blood sugar control mechanisms can eat whole foods sweetened with moderate amounts of honey or maple syrup and eat plenty of whole-grain foods without difficulty. This is not the case for most hypoglycemics. They have to use protein and fat to maintain normal blood sugar levels and not just three meals a day either. They require three moderate whole-food, unprocessed-carbohydrate meals a day with plenty of high-protein snacks between meals and before bed. (For a sample one-day meal plan, see page 92.) Regular intake of protein foods will prevent many of the symptoms of hypoglycemia for up to three to six hours. Combined with vitamin, mineral, and herbal supplementation with special emphasis on nutrients such as magnesium and GTF to correct dysfunctional metabolism, this diet can be extremely effective in eliminating the depression that is caused by functional hypoglycemia.

Sample One-Day Meal Plan for Stabilizing Blood Sugar

BREAKFAST

1/2 cup oatmeal with plain soy milk
Blueberry leaf herbal tea or coffee substitute
8 ounces nonfat yogurt (plain or flavored)

SNACK

High-protein, low-sugar energy bar

LUNCH

6 ounces pine nut tabbouleh
1 cup steamed sea vegetable (arame, wakamae, kombu, hijiki, nori)
1 medium tomato, sliced
1 cup romaine lettuce with natural dressing
1 medium apple
Blueberry leaf herbal tea or coffee substitute

SNACK

Marinated tofu

DINNER

6 ounces baked curry tempeh
1/2 cup steamed green peas
2 cups romaine lettuce and alfalfa sprouts with mustard dill dressing
6 ounces baked apple
Blueberry leaf herbal tea or coffee substitute

Nutritional Supplements for Hypoglycemia-Based Depression

A typical basic nutritional supplementation program for hypoglycemia might include 200 international units of vitamin E, 500 milligrams of vitamin C (ascorbic acid), a B-complex tablet, and individual
doses of other B vitamins including 100 milligrams of vitamin B_6, 500
milligrams of vitamin B_3, and 100 milligrams of pantothenic acid. For the

vitamin B_3, use niacinamide rather than niacin because some individuals experience nausea, itching, and flushing of the skin from niacin. After a few weeks the niacinamide and vitamin C dosage can be increased to 3,000 milligrams per day (1,000 milligrams after the morning, afternoon, and evening meals).

Low-Glycemic-Index Foods for Hypoglycemia

The organization of the glycemic index revolves around the ranking of glucose at an arbitrary figure of 100. Foods are evaluated according to how fast they turn into blood sugar (glucose) in comparison to sucrose. Foods with a glycemic index of above 100 turn into blood sugar even faster than sucrose. The higher the ranking of the food, the more glycemic it is. A food whose glycemic ranking is over 60 is considered high on the glycemic index. The higher a food ranks on the glycemic index, the greater its influence on glucose levels and the greater its potential to affect mood swings and other psychological symptoms. Keep in mind, however, that the impact a food will have on the blood sugar also depends on many other factors, such as the time of day the food is eaten, the length of time it was cooked, its fat content, its fiber levels, and its ripeness, as well as the activity just engaged in by the person eating the food and the person's insulin levels.

The best foods to use for stabilizing blood sugar based on the glycemic index are green leafy vegetables. Among the starchy vegetables, sweet potatoes (54) and green peas (48) are best. Fruits tend to be high on the glycemic index; however, those fruits that are lower and can be used in small amounts include grapes (43), oranges (43), peaches (42), pears (36), apples (36), plums (24), and cherries (22). With the exception of split peas (high on the glycemic index, with a rating of 82), most legumes are in the 30 to 49 range. However, soybeans are only 18, and peanuts are 14.

The best whole grains to use in a hypoglycemia-control diet are rolled oats and oatmeal (49), bulger (47), wheat kernels (41), hominy (40), whole wheat (37), puffed wheat (25), barley (25), and rice bran (19).

Foods with a ranking of under 45 are considered low on the glycemic index. They include beans; cruciferous vegetables such as cauliflower and broccoli; high-fiber, low-sugar cereals; low-fat, unsweetened plain yogurt; grapefruit; apples; and tomatoes.

I have found that the most effective approach to integrating the glycemic rating system with an herbal-based emotional healing system is to:

- Mix 30 percent of total calories from vegetarian proteins with 40 to 50 percent from carbohydrates ranked low to moderate on the glycemic index.
- Keep fat calories in the 20 to 25 percent range and get them from monounsaturates such as olive oil.
- Choose whole-grain breakfast cereals based on wheat bran, barley, and oats.
- Use whole-grain breads made with whole seeds.
- Use lemon juice and vinegar dressings.

In addition to the above, pay attention to portion control.

Alternative Tips for Hypoglycemia

In addition to maintaining a balanced diet of low-glycemic-index foods and using the appropriate supplements, you may wish to use essential oils, especially those scents and aromas that will reduce your desire to eat sweets. The aromas that serve hypoglycemics best are the scents of nutmeg, allspice, and cocoa butter.

Since craving sweets may actually be our body's way of trying to boost serotonin levels (the neurotransmitters linked with sweet cravings), anything that can boost serotonin may actually reduce these cravings. It is interesting to note that the drug Prozac also increases serotonin levels in the body. Many individuals taking Prozac for the treatment of depression find that their appetite and their craving for sweets are reduced.

Estrogen and Progesterone Imbalances

Estrogen is the basic female sex hormone produced by the body and is responsible for the development of female characteristics. Both men and women possess certain levels of what are called female and male hormones. However, women possess greater levels of estrogen than men. Estrogen is a potent and potentially dangerous hormone. The risk factors associated with it arise when it is not balanced by adequate levels of progesterone. In a healthy individual with balanced glandular function, progesterone is manufactured by the adrenal glands in men and women and in the ovaries in women. In pregnancy, the placenta will manufacture additional amounts.

Progesterone is a steroid hormone produced by the corpus luteum of the ovary at ovulation and also in the adrenal glands from the steroid hormone pregnenolone. Progesterone is a precursor to most of the other steroid hormones, including cortisol, the estrogens, and testosterone.

Recent research has also shown that the increased stress of a modern lifestyle, combined with a diet rich in highly processed, nutrient-depleted foods, has reduced levels of all female hormones, but especially progesterone. Though many physicians are aware of this problem, they often try to solve it by prescribing synthetic compounds known as progestins to treat the condition. Progestins were created to mimic the role of natural progesterone. However, over the years they have been found to produce many unpleasant side effects. Similar problems have arisen with xeno-estrogens, which are synthetic compounds that are environmental pollutants. Xenoestrogens occur as waste products of petrochemical-based industries. When our bodies are exposed to these agents, or we ingest them, they act like estrogen and may have the same or similar negative effects as occur with the unopposed synthetic estrogen that is often prescribed by physicians.

In recent years it has become a common practice for physicians to prescribe the hormone estrogen for women with menopausal symptoms. It is believed that by doing so they can replace the hormones lost with the advent of menopause. Contemporary physicians now know that estrogen replacement therapy (ERT) is not a desirable procedure and that it is not estrogen that needs to be replaced but rather another hormone, progesterone. In fact, a cause of many health problems associated with PMS and menopause, including depression, hypgolycemia, mood swings, and thyroid deficiency, is a condition known as *estrogen dominance*. This condition results when the normal ratio or balance of the hormones estrogen and progesterone is shifted by an excess of estrogen or inadequate amounts of progesterone.

The synthetic progestins generally prescribed by doctors in hormone replacement therapy are not progesterone, and do not actually replace the body's progesterone in any biochemically equal form. In fact, fertility specialists cannot use synthetic progestins in their work.

Natural hormone replacement therapy (NHRT), on the other hand, utilizes hormones that are biochemically identical to those hormones manufactured by a woman's body. When NHRT is used in creating hormonal balance in the body, many menopausal symptoms disappear as well as the depression, weight gain, irritability, increased risk of breast cancer, and other side effects associated with menopause.

One of the benefits of natural progesterone is that it opposes or balances the effects of estrogen. As a woman ages, her estrogen levels will drop as much as 40 to 60 percent, leading to menopause and the cessation of her menstrual cycle. In some women, however, progesterone levels may drop to nearly zero. Since progesterone is a precursor to many other steroid hormones, its use can greatly improve overall hormone balance after menopause. This rebalancing of the estrogen-progesterone ratio may also stimulate bone building and thus help protect against osteoporosis and reduce the risk of breast cancer, reproductive cancers, and hormone-based depression.

Progesterone Cream

One of the most effective ways to balance hormonal levels is through the use of plant-derived progesterone cream with phytoestrogens or a plant-derived progesterone cream without phytoestrogens. The latter is best for men, a breast-feeding woman, or a pregnant woman. Phytoestrogen herbs are beneficial for helping to keep your estrogen levels from elevating to an unhealthy level. According to Dr. John Lee, an expert on the use of progesterone, the best cream to use is one that has 450 to 500 milligrams of USP progesterone per ounce, which is 1.6 percent by weight or 3 percent by volume.

According to Dr. John Lee:

> The USP progesterone used for hormone replacement comes from plant fats and oils, usually a substance called diosgenin which is extracted from a very specific type of wild yam that grows in Mexico, or from soybeans. In the laboratory diosgenin is chemically synthesized into real human progesterone. The other human steroid hormones, including estrogen, testosterone, and the cortisones, are also nearly always synthesized from diosgenin.[2]

USP progesterone is the type of progesterone that you want to be using for hormone replacement.

There are generally three types of plant-based hormone delivery systems; these are capsules and tablets, vaginal suppositories, and creams. Respected experts on the use of progesterone have differing points of view of each. Speak with a nutritional consultant or holistic physician familiar with the estrogen-progesterone issue as it relates to depression to see which is most appropriate for your needs.

Though I have avoided mentioning particular brands, physicians, or laboratories, most of the experts on progesterone supplementation and the testing of saliva and general glandular function have mentioned various laboratories as a source for cutting-edge diagnostic approaches to depression, especially thyroid, adrenal, and progesterone testing. Diagnos-Techs, Inc., was established in 1987 and was the first lab in the United States to implement salivary-based hormone assessment into routine clinical practice. For further information, they can be contacted at Diagnos-Techs, Inc., 6620 South 192nd Place, Building J, Kent, WA 98032; (800) 878-3787.

Precautions

Hormone products, whether synthetic or natural, are the source of much confusion and controversy. There are many different products available, as well as contradictory views among the experts concerning which are best and how to use them most effectively. The experts with whom I spoke on this subject have long histories in the field of holistic nutrition and alternative medicine, and they have been helpful to me over the years in clarifying other issues in health and healing. They believe that taking estrogen or progesterone is key for relieving many types of depression, but add that anyone who takes a hormone product needs to keep the following precautions in mind.

- Avoid progesterone creams that contain the herb licorice if you have hypertension. There have been a few reports that licorice can slightly raise blood pressure in some individuals.
- Do not use natural progesterone cream if you are taking birth control pills. Because birth control pills contain synthetic progestins, which attach to the progesterone receptor sites in the body, much of the natural progesterone contained in the cream will not be able to attach to these receptors, thus preventing you from getting much benefit from it. In addition, the natural progesterone might upset the hormone balance in the birth control pills and interfere with their contraceptive benefits.
- Though progesterone cream can be used safely with most medications, it is always beneficial to check with a nutritionally aware

physician before starting any new high-dosage supplement or hormone product.

- The use of natural progestrone is generally free of side effects and there are no reports of any other significant health problems with these plant hormones. However, the *Physicians' Desk Reference*, an annual guide to all the medications available, does offer a long list of side effects and contraindications for synthetic hormones generally referred to as progesterone. These are different products than plant-based progesterone.

- It is beneficial to check progesterone levels by means of a saliva test the first few months to adjust dosage. Hormonal needs may vary month to month and you want to avoid taking too much or too little. Though some physicians use a combination of serum and saliva testing to determine appropriate hormone levels, only the saliva test is accurate for progesterone. This is because progesterone, being fat-soluble, cannot be effectively tested through blood testing, which is best suited for water-soluble blood components. Natural progesterone is fat-soluble (carried by fat-soluble red blood cells), and thus easily absorbed through the skin, especially at areas rich with capillaries. These are generally located at those areas of the skin where people blush: palms of hands, face, inner armpits, breasts, and chest. In these areas the hormone is absorbed into the blood circulation. Since there are fluctuations in progesterone levels, these should be tested only using a saliva hormone radioimmunoassay (RIA).

- One of the problems with progesterone supplementation for depression is that the most common side effect of excessive progesterone use is depression. Therefore, it is key that you determine the most appropriate dose for you.

If you are being treated with products such as Premarin, Provera, and PremPro, you may want to explore replacing these with NHRT. If you are going to explore this approach to improving your health, it is best to consult with a supportive physician, a nutritional consultant, or a knowledgeable pharmacist.

Thyroid Disorders

Dr. Broda Barnes, a pioneering researcher on thyroid function, showed that many infections (especially those of the respiratory tract such as tonsillitis, sore throats, sinusitis, pneumonia, and middle ear infections) can be eliminated when the body's thyroid levels are normal.

It is known that behavior, mood, and cognitive function can be affected by changes in thyroid function. Recent research suggests that thyroid disorders are among the most common physical problems that contribute to depression. In fact, some individuals might have subclinical hypothyroidism (underactive thyroid gland function) that produces few if any symptoms other than depression. Treatment of this condition may be all that's required to cure chronic depression.

There is a clear connection between the process of thyroid hormone regulation and bipolar disorder. This connection, however, is only just now beginning to become evident. Is that because the thyroid problems somehow actually cause bipolar-like symptoms? Could it be that some of what looks like a bipolar disorder is actually a thyroid problem? In many cases, bipolar symptoms get better when thyroid hormones are part of the treatment.

An article in the *Journal of Clinical Psychiatry* shows that the thyroid hormone T3 can be used to treat post-traumatic stress disorder, commonly seen in soldiers and people who have been through other causes of terrible emotional trauma.[3]

A study conducted in 1998 indicates that certain depressions may be a response to an underactive thyroid, even when no symptoms of hypothyroidism are apparent. The study by Im Jackson, published in the journal *Thyroid*, states in part, "It is known that in human depression there is a functional disconnection of the hypothalamus with impairment of the inhibitory glucocorticoid feedback pathway from the hippocampus to the hypothalamus that results in the typical elevated cortisol levels and impaired dexamethasone suppression."[4]

The thyroid gland is important to mental health because it increases enzymes that affect the metabolic rate of brain cells as well as stimulating particular regions of the brain. Many researchers believe that the link between hypothyroidism and depression is the oxygen supply to the brain.

Hypothyroidism is one of the most common and generally undiagnosed causes of depression. In 1976, I attended a lecture by Dr. Broda

Barnes, who stated that in as early as the 1940s, he saw that blood tests used to determine thyroid activity in patients were often inaccurate. Many patients with low thyroid activity, when tested, might produce blood readings on the thyroid hormones T3, T4, T7, and thyroid stimulating hormone (TSH) that might be considered within "normal" ranges and still suffer from underactive thyroid. According to Dr. Barnes, who published more than a hundred papers and several books on the thyroid gland and its influence in human health, as much as 40 percent of the adult U.S. population was affected by this condition. Dr. Barnes's writings describe a situation where individuals often suffered from symptoms that might include depression, mental sluggishness, confusion, fatigue, low sex drive, brittle hair, puffiness around the eyes, cold hands and feet, sleeping more than eight hours a night, susceptibility to colds and infections, slow weight loss, loss of memory, poor concentration, obesity, migraine headaches, infertility, menstrual problems, skin problems (including acne and dryness), thinning hair, hypertension, atherosclerosis, and blood sugar metabolism problems (including diabetes and hypoglycemia).

Many individuals who experience these symptoms may have low thyroid function as the cause and yet traditional medical tests will indicate that these patients have normal thyroid function. When these same individuals were given thyroid replacement therapy, many or all of these symptoms disappeared.

The situation has not changed much since Dr. Barnes's discovery in the 1940s. It is only in recent years that new thyroid tests have been developed to give physicians and patients accurate readings of thyroid function. Most of these tests focus on T3 levels as the most important indicator of thyroid balance.

Since selenium is essential for synthesis, activation, and metabolism of thyroid hormone, it seems natural that the level of selenium in the body might influence thyroid function. Selenium levels, especially selenium deficiency, most likely influence psychological health, including behavior, mood, and cognitive function. Though it is often difficult to isolate a specific hormonal factor as a cause of depression, there are a number of health problems associated with thyroid function including decreased immune function, especially increased susceptibility to viral infections. When these thyroid deficiency symptoms arise, it is important to look at selenium deficiency as a key factor.

New technologies now enable doctors to achieve more accurate measurements of biologically active thyroid hormones from saliva specimens. A recently developed test, the fluorescence activated microsphere assay (available from ImmunoDiagnostic Laboratories in San Leandro, California), should be done as well. This test can reveal abnormalities that older medical tests often missed.

Thyroid function can also be evaluated through a simple blood test called the TSH test. This test is so accurate that it can determine whether a person is suffering from an overactive or underactive thyroid often before the patient begins to experience symptoms.

New guidelines have been established for physicians testing for thyroid function. Doctors are encouraged to consider thyroid treatment for patients who test within the TSH range of 0.3 to 3.04, a far narrower range than what was considered problematic before. It is believed that the new guidelines may actually double the number of people who have abnormal thyroid function (bringing the total to as many as 27 million) and may help many patients who would otherwise be misdiagnosed.

Activating Your Thyroid

Most mainstream physicians recommend synthetic thyroid to stimulate an underactive thyroid. This, however, should not be the first course of action unless you are in a critical situation. There are a number of ways of gently stimulating thyroid activity. If tests indicate that hyperthyroidism is the source of your symptoms, speak with a nutritionally based or holistic physician; however, there are products available that are more balanced in the spectrum of factors they contain.

Herbs That Gently Stimulate Thyroid Activity

Sea vegetables are useful for optimizing thyroid function—especially low thyroid—and for regulating the immune system. Irish moss, dulse, and kelp are good sources of calcium, magnesium, sodium, and naturally occurring lithium and iodine (essential to normal thyroid function). They are used to increase the metabolic rate. These sea vegetables also contain mucilaginous compounds that enhance the detoxifying and eliminative functions of the digestive system.

Other thyroid-balancing factors include spirulina algae and the herbs black cohosh (an excellent all-round female tonifier except during pregnancy), valerian, passion flower, hops, licorice root (good for boosting adrenal function), and milk thistle (silymarin, an additional antioxidant and liver cleanser).

If these are not effective in reducing your symptoms, then speak with a nutritionally based or holistic physician. Dr. Barnes treated thyroid disorders with natural desiccated thyroid rather than synthetic thyroid preparations like Synthroid. The advantage of natural thyroid over synthetic is that with the former the body's own deficient thyroid hormones are replaced with the natural product, whereas synthetics do not duplicate all of the subtle aspects of this hormone.

Thyroid hormone has also been shown to sometimes be a treatment for bipolar disorder. Thyroid hormones can act as a mood treatment, even when a person's thyroid levels seem to be "normal." In some individuals, these hormones, given in addition to the person's usual production, change something in the brain that affects mood. In at least some cases, thyroid hormones are a treatment for mood problems that aren't thyroid problems in the first place.

According to some experts, the combination of T3 and T4 seems to act much more powerfully and consistently than either one alone. In some cases, they have been reported to act in a similar manner as lithium. Speak to your physician for the most appropriate choice for you.

For sources of further information on thyroid issues relating to depression and other symptoms, see "Resources" on page 224.

Candida and Lowered Immunity

Lowered immunity can lead to depression such as occurs with certain types of yeast infections, and depression can affect immunity as well. According to Lynanne McGuire, Ph.D., of the Johns Hopkins School of Medicine, the lead author of an article published in the *Journal of Abnormal Psychology*, "Depressive symptoms can exacerbate and accelerate the immunological declines that typically accompany aging."[5]

It has been known for many years that the brain, nervous system, endocrine system, and immune system regulate one another's functioning. Studies show that the immune system is compromised by prolonged depression, and recovery is slowed from many medical conditions. This is especially risky for those over sixty-five years of age, who have a greater risk of infection and injuries, especially broken hips. This slowed rate of recovery can, in turn, worsen the depression, creating a vicious downward emotional and physical spiral.

The premature death of brain cells in diseases such as amyotrophic lateral sclerosis (ALS), better known as Lou Gehrig's disease; Alzheimer's disease; and Parkinson's disease; is linked to a progressive collapse of the immune system. This dialogue between your brain and your immune system depends on two chemical languages, the brain's neurotransmitters and the immune system's immunotransmitters. An area of the brain known as the hypothalamus monitors this biological interaction. The hypothalamus connects your brain to various systems in the body, including your breathing, energy balance, heat regulation, nervous system, endocrine system, immune system, circulatory system, and emotions (moods).

Candida and Depression

Any health problem that reduces immunity or negatively affects your glandular system can contribute to brain-related disorders, including depression. One connection between immunity and depression became apparent when individuals suffering from bipolar disorder reported reduction of some of their symptoms from antifungal therapy. This pointed researchers to yeast, a type of fungus, as a possible causative factor.

Evidence suggests that one type of naturally occurring yeast, called candida, may overgrow in certain conditions and may activate depressive symptoms and other health problems by promoting ethanol production, a known central nervous system depressant. Yeast overgrowth may also come about in response to a weakened immune system.

A compromised immune system can lead to an extreme overgrowth of *Candida albicans*. Many in the holistic and alternative medicine community believe that this *Candida albicans* hypersensitivity, also called chronic disseminated candidiasis or candidiasis (*can di DI a sis*), is a major cause of a host of emotional and physical problems. Yeast overgrowth usually results from thyroid and endocrine dysfunction, antibiotic use, stress, and overconsumption of refined carbohydrates and alcohol. It can be diagnosed by laboratory testing.

Many of the symptoms associated with candida are also common to many other medical problems including low blood sugar, glandular imbalances, various subclinical nutrition deficiencies, and various allergies. Allergic symptoms are also influenced by many variables, including mood shifts. It would be extremely difficult to design a controlled study that would separate these variables and present a concise statement on what level of candida causes what symptoms.

The concept of candidiasis hypersensitivity was first publicly articulated by C. Orian Truss, M.D., of Birmingham, Alabama, and expanded upon by William G. Crook, M.D., of Jackson, Tennessee. Some proponents suggest that chronic fatigue syndrome is closely related to candida infections.

Diagnosing Candida

It is difficult to make a specific diagnosis of candida; thus, the most conservative approach would be to avoid assuming you have the disorder without definite clinical signs of a local infection. These may include a discharge, rash, itching, or soreness.

Some nutritionists and physicians use what is called the comprehensive digestive stool analysis (CDSA). This test evaluates digestion, absorption, intestinal function, and the type and quality of bacteria in the intestines. The test results may reveal possible causes and contributing factors to the onset of depression.

Candida symptoms alone are not the most effective way to diagnose candida overgrowth. Serious intestinal candidiasis is a well-documented problem. The only true way to diagnose candida is to take a biopsy of the intestine with an instrument called an endoscope. This test can be performed by a gastroenterologist. It is an invasive procedure and is not recommended unless your depression is so extreme that it inhibits your ability to function and no other factor seems to be the cause.

Treating Candida

When treating candidiasis, the goal is to remove the yeast from the infected tissue, return yeast levels to normal in the body, and rebuild the immune system. In the early days of candida research, it was believed by many that eliminating most fermented foods and any fungus- and yeast-containing foods from the diet was the most effective approach to reducing yeast overgrowth. At that time it was believed that these foods increased candida growth. Research in recent years has shown that certain mushrooms including shiitake (*Lentinus edodes*) actually contain a potent antifungal agent that is effective against *Candida albicans*. Shiitake—the most popular edible mushroom used in most Asian cuisine, especially in Japan and China—contains a variety of constituents that have demonstrated a range of actions, including immune modulation. Its bioactive constituents include beta-glucan, heteroglucan, adenine derivative, guanosine 5'-mono-phosphate, and polyacelylene. Reports indicate that this fungus is most effective against candida when taken in extract form.

The Link Between Candida and Other Problems

Individuals with low gastric acidity may also experience increased levels of depression through a candida connection. Low gastric activity may lead to a bacterial overgrowth in the small intestine, which in turn interferes with protein digestion. With reduced absorption of protein comes reduced availability of key pathways for important amino acids.

The links between low blood sugar and candidiasis are also strong. A diet of high-glycemic foods will aggravate the symptoms of hypoglycemia and also tend to increase growth of *Candida albicans*. In individuals who suffer from both low blood sugar and weakened immunity, the effects can be devastating, with their depression originating from related but different causes. For such individuals a therapeutic program has to address many variables at the same time without overwhelming the patient. Any program needs to be based on each individual's history and response to treatment. With this in mind, the following is a long-term program to help your body detoxify the chronic infection.

The thirteen steps should be started one at a time. A few days after starting one step, start the next. If you are very ill now, start slowly and work up.

1. Take steps to normalize your bowel movements. It is important to have two bowel movements per day. Candida affects the small intestine (causing fermentation, gas, bloating, and reflux) and often begins with chronic constipation. Do not start this detoxification program until your bowels are working every day.
2. Increase your use of high-fiber foods and herbs to help maintain the entire gastrointestinal system and keep it functioning properly, while promoting healthful bacteria. One benefit of high-fiber intestinal-cleansing herbs and foods is that they help loosen the tough mucus that candida will form on the intestinal wall, helping to remove it from the body and improving the absorption

of important vitamins and minerals. Cleansing products include bentonite, psyllium seed husks, citrus pectin, organic wheat grass, cascara sagrada, buckthorn, goldenseal, and black walnut husks. Purchase a basic anticandida formula designed to help reduce the infection count in the bowels.

3. Discontinue any antibiotics or steriods you may be using, unless they are absolutely necessary. Antibiotics promote the growth of yeast in the body and can destroy intestinal microflora.

4. Replace intestinal microflora by using a probiotic formula containing pharmaceutical-grade acidophilus and bifidus to assist the intestines in lowering the candida infection.

5. Use colloidal silver, which kills certain bacteria and viruses, fights candida, and heals injured tissues. To one glass of the tea or any full glass of liquid, add a half-teaspoon of colloidal silver, 500 ppm, twice daily for sixty days. Then reduce to once a day for another sixty days.

6. Take oregano capsules, which are especially helpful if there is severe gas or bloating after eating a large meal. There are a number of products available that combine oregano oil, ginger oil, and fennel oil. Take oregano oil in doses of 0.2 to 0.4 milliliters twice a day. Do not overuse oregano oil since it can be dangerous in high doses.

7. Use nutritional supplements that have been shown to increase and balance the function of the immune system. Supplements that have antioxidant properties and immunity-boosting qualities include acidophilus, evening primrose oil, vitamin E, linseed oil, caprylic acid, and pau d'arco. Pau d'arco (taheebo) is available in tea form or liquid extract and is highly effective against candida and other fungal infections. Apparently components of the herb penetrate into body tissues and work on a cellular level. Also use fresh garlic (one raw bulb daily) plus an aged garlic supplement (4 grams daily) for four weeks.

8. Use an antiparasitic herbal combination. A popular formula consists of pumpkin, marshmallow root, culvers root, cascara sagrada bark, mullein leaves, chamomile flowers, violet leaves, and slippery elm bark. This formula not only eliminates parasites but supports the immune system as well. A classic Western herbal formula for boosting the number of immune cells and other important natural immune chemicals in the blood consists of echinacea, Siberian

ginseng, pau d'arco, astragalus, olive leaf, and garlic. This formula is also helpful for shortening the duration of existing infections and providing greater resistance against future infections. Another effective herbal formula to reduce candida overgrowth contains lapacho, an immunostimulant; barberry, an antinflammatory good for digestive disorders; marigold, an antifungal; echinacea, an immunostimulant; bladderwrack, a sea vegetable; and galangal, an immunostimulant. All are effective against candida and some bacteria.

9. Eliminate caffeine. The caffeine in one cup of coffee can kill up to 75 percent of the friendly acidophilus flora in the colon.

10. Take nutritional supplements that build up the body's immunity and kill off the yeast or make it difficult for it to reproduce. Three of the most powerful immune builders are selenium, olive leaf extract, and bovine colustrum.

11. Eat a low-carbohydrate diet. Because yeast feeds on sugar, wheat, and dairy products, they should be avoided. Yeasts, molds, and fungi crossreact so avoid yeast products such as alcohol, vinegar, most mushrooms, commercial breads, and cheeses.

12. Discontinue your use of birth control pills, especially if you have a discharge or headaches with your monthly periods. The progestins in these pills cause changes in the vaginal mucous membrane, which makes it easier for candida to multiply. Because of this, you may need to avoid natural progesterone products as well. First you must determine if it is candida or low progesterone that is the primary cause of your depression.

13. Consider taking the antifungal drug nystatin. When nothing seems to help, some doctors prescribe nystatin, which is effective only in the digestive tract. Consider purchasing enteric-coated softgels for maximum delivery if you experience throat or stomach upset and reflux.

Whatever road you take with your candida treatment, remember that it will take an average of six to twelve months to irradicate candida overgrowth even if your treatment is persistent. The initial symptoms to improve will be diarrhea, headaches, chemical sensitivities, vaginitis, and emotional and behavior problems.

Other individual herbs and nutritional factors that are known to reduce candida growth include barberry, *Echinacea purpurea*, garlic, betaine hydrochloride, goldenseal, caprylic acid, oregano oil, enzymes, *Lactobacillus acidophilus,* Oregon grape, peppermint oil, rosemary oil, tea tree oil, and thyme oil.

Caprylic acid (a naturally occurring fatty acid) is an effective antifungal compound against candida infections of the intestines. Doctors often recommend amounts of 500 to 1,000 milligrams three times a day.

Though there is more research on the value of nutritional supplements than ever before, medical culture as a whole does not lean toward the use of supplements to treat medical problems. Until just a few years ago, much of the information available about nutrition and the treatment of disease was based on preliminary research and anecdotal information.

If you try the supplements recommended in this chapter, use them in moderation; do not take unnecessarily large doses. In addition, remember to integrate your nutritional program with herbs, aromatherapy, and other healing tools discussed in this book.

6 ❧ REDUCING DEPRESSION WITH AROMATHERAPY

A good part of any person's emotional well-being is determined by how he or she responds to the surrounding environment. Smell is a key factor in most forms of human activity, particularly that which is necessary for social interaction. Many societies use the scent produced by incense in ritual and religious practice. Combined with repetition, chanting, singing, and prayer, a familiar scent can have a powerful influence on an individual or a group. This is, in part, because the aroma functions primarily on a subliminal or subconscious level. The aroma and what an individual or community associates with it may have a direct impact on the emotional centers of the brain without the interference of intellectual or rational thought. These are issues that are still to be addressed as having importance in culturally specific depression.

Aromatherapy is the therapeutic use of the scents produced by essential oils. These oils are extracted from the flower, leaf, stalk, or fruit of a plant, shrub, or tree. A pleasant aroma can connect us to a warm deep, content, safe place within ourselves. No one looks forward to being presented with an unpleasant odor. It is for this very reason that cosmetic, food, and pharmaceutical companies place great importance on specific aromas in certain products. Menthol scent is often used in chest rubs and cough drops, lemon is added to many cleaning products, and cosmetic companies invest millions in associating various perfumes and colognes with current celebrities.

The powerful sense of smell and the impact of "aromas" on physical and psychological states can be exemplified by the extreme physical reactions such as "gagging" or "heaving" that we experience when coming in contact with a particularly offensive smell.

As adults, many of us have been taught that expressing our emotions is unacceptable, so when looking for comfort, we may seek out something that brings back the memory of a pleasant aroma from childhood: maybe a special food, candy, or some specific environment. Our brains associate the memory brought on by an aroma with the relief of emotional stress.

The History of Aromatherapy

Giovanni Gatti and Renato Cayola conducted the earliest scientific investigation of the power of aroma to influence emotions and the nervous system in the early 1920s. These Italian physicians published a report, "The Action of Essences on the Nervous System," which explored the effects of different essential oils on anxiety and depression. After exposing study subjects to oils taken both orally and through inhalation, they measured changes in their blood circulation, pulse rate, and depth of breathing.

Their results showed for the first time that scents could quickly influence the brain. The study also showed clearly that inhalation of the aromatic oils brought about a much quicker effect than oral administration. Clearly the oils entered the system at a quicker rate when inhaled than through the slower absorptive process of the digestive system. Drs. Gatti and Cayola made note of which oils seemed to have the greatest influence on what we would now classify as manic or depressive patterns. The essential oils that they identified as sedatives, and most useful for reducing anxiety-based, manic behavior, included asafetida, chamomile, melissa, neroli, opoponax, petitgrain, and valerian. The oils they identified as stimulating, best for the treatment of depression, included angelica, cardamom, fennel, and lemon. In addition, they discovered, to their surprise, that some essences, though stimulating in smaller doses, were sedating when used in larger amounts. The researchers concluded that "the sense of smell has, by reflex action, an enormous influence on the function of the central nervous system."[1]

The term *aromatherapy* was coined in 1937 in Rene-Maurice Gattefosse's classic work *Aromatherapie*, and much research on oils had been conducted since then.

Apparently the best approach to aromatherapy involves creating a pleasant-smelling blend of different oils. Combinations of oils bring different therapeutic properties to the process and also tend to have a more pleasant aroma than individual oils. Interestingly the scents we associate with food as well as the scents of aromatic oils stimulate the part of the brain that is responsible for feelings of both discomfort and well-being (the limbic area). It is for this reason that great interest has focused on the inhalation of plant oils as an alternative to antidepressant medication.

Various researchers have found the aromatic oils of lemon, orange, verbena, jasmine, ylang-ylang, and sandalwood to be most effective against the symptoms of depression. Among the anxiety-relieving oils that these researchers have found to be effective were bergamot, lavender, lime, neroli, and petitgrain.

In the 1970s, Professor Torii of Toho University, Japan, created a research program with the aim of specifically defining those oils possessing a sedative effect on the nervous system and those with a stimulating effect. Using an electroencephalogram (EEG), a test that measures brain waves, and a measuring device called a contingent negative variation (CNV) curve, an electrical brain wave pattern was created. According to the results, lavender had a sedative effect on the nervous system and jasmine a stimulating one.

Interestingly Professor Torii also found in further research that certain oils (specifically geranium and rosewood and less so valerian) could be either stimulating or sedating, depending on the state of the individual. This unusual quality is known by herbalists as an "adaptogen" effect. This effect is common with various herbs, including Siberian ginseng. Adaptogens produce a balancing effect, essentially restorative for depressed patients as well as those who are manic, agitated, or prone to hyperactivity. Much more important work has been done over the years on the effect of aromatic oils on the brain.

Aromatherapy, the Brain, and the Emotions

Research conducted on the emotions and brain function during olfactory stimulation on the left and right sides of the brain has determined that out of all the senses, smell is the only one processed in the emotional, creative, right side of the brain. Simply speaking, the right-hand side controls aesthetic awareness, imagination, and the emotions while the left-hand side controls logic, reasoning, and words. Under normal circumstances both sides of the brain function in harmony, integrating information from the various senses. However, researchers discovered that when a subject inhaled a perfume described as "pleasant," intense electrical activity took place in the right hemisphere. In time as the brain was able to integrate this olfactory stimulus, the activity spread to parts of the left hemisphere as well. These researchers also discovered that during the perception of an odor, the cognitive part (left hemisphere) of the brain could block an emotional reaction (taking place in the right hemisphere of the brain) if it determined that such a response was inappropriate. The left hemisphere was even able to completely block out a hedonistic experience [2]

As you can see, brain wave activity is a complex affair, and even though certain aromas are prone to be stimulating or sedating when used therapeutically, the effect of an aroma on an individual may ultimately depend on the emotional state or mental attitude of the patient. This does not apply simply to aromatherapy. Clearly, aromatherapy is a valid therapeutic tool that goes beyond placebo affect and still it must be acknowledged that in certain situations subjective psychological factors can influence and even dominate an objective physiological reaction.

It is for this reason that a holistic, integrative approach to the treatment of depression is so important, even when a person requires medication. Visualization, meditation, cognitive behavioral therapy, tai chi, yoga, and a multitude of other approaches build off each other to create a mental-emotional environment for the individual that will maximize the benefits of the essential oil.

The limbic system, the emotional "control center" of the brain, is greatly influenced by aromas. Thus it is possible to greatly influence a patient's attitude or disposition through aromatherapy. It is not just the biochemical quality of the scent that counts. If a depressed individual has a positive association with a specific scent, that scent can be integrated into a meditation or visualization exercise, possibly resulting in a remembrance of a time of happiness, joy, and contentment and an opportunity to reexperience those emotions.

Odors are processed in the emotional center of our brains because these scents are necessary for our survival. Not only do we react to the smell of cut roses or our mom's casserole, but we also respond to odors we don't consciously detect such as pheromones, odorous substances that abound in the human and animal world. It is believed that these scents were responsible for man's early survival and, through the years, have been replaced by our reliance on vision. Some depressed individuals, especially those who suffer from hypoglycemia or zinc deficiency, may experience a loss of the sense of smell. People with weight problems will sometimes complain that they see food and are then hungry, when the truth really is that they detect the odor of the food and then have the conditioned response to eat or not eat, depending on whether they like the smell or not. Smell, clearly, is part of our primal history.

Over the last few years important research has been conducted on the effect of aromatic oils on the brain. In 1979, John Steele began evaluating the effects of various essential oils on the brain's rhythmic patterns. He discovered that antidepressant euphorics such as jasmine, rose, and neroli oils induced an unusual amount of delta brain waves with some alpha and theta brain waves as well. Stress management experts, biofeedback technicians, and clinical hypnotherapists know that slower frequencies of this type indicate a quieting of unfocused mental activity, with an increase in intuitive flashes and a sense of recovery.

There are three mechanisms through which smell affects our emotions, moods, and physiology:

1. **Psychological.** This is the initial reaction that most of us have to a particular smell or aroma. This may include memories associated with a particular scent and contextual association.
2. **Pharmacological.** This is essentially the intrinsic pharmacological property of the odor molecule itself on various areas of the brain.
3. **Physiological.** This is the general effect a particular oil has on the body. In most cases this is a sedating or a stimulating effect. This effect can be greatly influenced by various factors, including the chemical reactions between the various enzymes and hormones in the bloodstream and the essential oil.

Much of the physiological effect associated with aromatic oils is based on the effect these oils have on the nervous system. For example, when we recognize the smell of an onion, what we are actually smelling is not just an odor but a reaction between an odor molecule and the stimulation of the trigeminal nerve found in the nose and face. Some people may experience a loss of the sense of smell owing to nerve damage or some other factor such as a zinc deficiency.

Studies show that people who lose their sense of smell are much more likely to develop generalized anxiety disorders. One popular theory states that just as there are sounds that we cannot hear, there also exist scents that are so subliminal that we are not aware they exist. Even these scents are capable of influencing human behavior. Thus those individuals who have lost the sense of smell may lose the benefit these subliminal scents offer as an integral part of mood regulation. For this reason, eating foods that stimulate the trigeminal nerve, such as peppermint, chili pepper, and horseradish, have been found to be helpful in restoring sensations.

Perhaps you've had the experience of fainting and having someone revive you with smelling salts. It happens because the trigeminal nerve is stimulated, which activates the part of the brain that keeps you awake. Tear gas has a similar effect in that burning eyes and difficulty in breathing are responses to an odor. In both cases it is an odor that stimulates a nerve.

Research on brain response to fragrance indicates that smells can influence mood, the production of hormones, memory, and even the immune system, all influential factors in the onset and healing of depression. In order to understand how these oils can affect physiology, alter moods, and heal the emotions, it is useful to understand the relationship between aromas, the glandular system, and brain response.

According to Alan R. Hirsch, M.D., the medical director of the Smell and Taste Treatment and Research Foundation, Chicago, Illinois, much of the effect of smell on how we act has to do with the hypothalamus, the part of the brain where many emotional drives are regulated.

In recent years there has been a groundswell in research concerning the aroma-recognizing mechanism in humans, and how the brain processes this information. Much of this research has been done by electrophysiologists, anatomists, psychologists, and most recently molecular biologists. One of the great breakthroughs in this research was in 1991, when researchers discovered that mammals are able to recognize odors by way of over a thousand distinct odor receptors located in the nerve tissue of the nasal cavity.

In several papers published in the mid-1990s in the journal *Cell*, Dr. Linda B. Buck and her colleagues at Harvard Medical School and Dr. Richard Axel and Dr. Robert Vassar and their co-workers at Columbia University College of Physicians and Surgeons in New York independently described the process by which odor receptors are distributed in the nose, and are connected to the smelling centers of the brain. These papers also describe how odor molecules traveling from the nostrils to olfactory membranes behind the bridge of the nose to the brain present information that is increasingly organized and refined.

How an individual reacts to a specific aroma is to a large part cultural, and age related. What is pleasant to one person may be unpleasant to another. There are few smells that people universally find to be pleasant or unpleasant. Even a person's career or hobby can influence how he or she reacts to a particular smell. For example, most of us find the sweet aroma of fresh-cut flowers to be extremely pleasant, but this may not be the case for people employed in the funeral business. They may associate this odor with death and decay. For some people, smell is a biochemical response, and for others, it is cultural. Whichever the case may be, aroma is a powerful healer for emotional trauma and depression.

The Four Emotions and the Categories of Oils

Every day we experience love and hate and an entire array of feelings, passions, sensibilities, and emotions. In order to be healthy, you must express them. Our ability to be in touch with and express our emotions plays a large part in the choices we make. Essential oils are a precious tool for naturally and easily getting in touch with and releasing locked feelings.

Plant essences act in two ways. Initially, the essence has either a soothing or an exciting effect on the nervous system. Your senses react to the aroma of the essence as you would to the aroma of perfume or a flower. In addition, the chemical composition of each individual essence has its own specific effect on the tissues and organs of the body.

Many emotional problems can be cared for with essential oils, particularly if they are detected and treated early. Essences can be classified according to function, including antispasmodics, antiseptics, stimulants, and sedatives. It is the stimulating and sedating oils that have the strongest effect on the emotions.

The stimulating oils include cardamon, cedar, cinnamon, fennel, lemon, and ylang-ylang. These are best when people experience a sense of immobility and are so depressed that they feel as if they can't even get out of bed.

The sedating oils include cajuput, chamomile, melissa, and peppermint. They are used to relieve insomnia and nervousness, and manic activity. Clinical studies of the psychological effects of chamomile oil, carried out recently at Cambridge University and the University of North Wales, confirmed the oil's soothing effect on the nervous system of humans.

For a list of oils that seem to reduce depression or help relieve the symptoms related to depression, see "Mental and Emotional Conditions and Aromatic Oils" below and on next page.

Many of the essential oils used for depression are from flowers or fruits. Aromatherapists report that any of the following oils may be used to combat depression: allspice, ambrette, basil, bergamot, Canadian balsam, cassie, cedarwood, clary sage, grapefruit, helichrysum, jasmine, lavender, melissa, neroli, orange, patchouli, rose, rosemary, rosewood, thyme, violet, and ylang-ylang.

Though you may experience almost immediate benefits from aromatherapy, a consistent stabilization of the symptoms of depression are difficult to achieve in less than a few months. Impatience and frustration can even aggravate the depression and make an individual irritated and anxiety-ridden. Be patient.

Mental and Emotional Conditions and Aromatic Oils

Certain aromatic oils have been found to work particularly well for depression in general and for its specific mental and emotional conditions.

ANGER	Ylang-ylang
ANXIETY	Bergamot*
	Bitter orange flower (neroli)
	Floral musk (labdanum)
	Frankincense
	Jasmine (absolute)
	Patchouli
	Rose (absolute)
	Vanilla
APATHY	Frankincense
	Jasmine (absolute)
	Mimos (absolute)
	Myrrh
	Tangerine
	Vetiver
DEPRESSION IN GENERAL	Bitter orange flower (neroli)
	Chamomile
	Frankincense

	Lavender
	Patchouli
	Rose (absolute)
	Sandlewood
	Tangerine
DISTURBING DREAMS	Mugwort
FEAR	Bitter orange flower (neroli)
FRUSTRATION	Ylang-ylang
GRIEF	Rose (absolute)
HYSTERIA	Bitter orange flower (neroli)
	Labdanum (floral musk)
	Lavender
	Vanilla
IMPOTENCE	Sandlewood
	Ylang-ylang
INSOMNIA	Cypress
	Lavender
	Roman chamomile
	Ylang-ylang
IRRITABILITY	Roman chamomile
RELATIONSHIP PROBLEMS	Jasmine (absolute)
SEXUAL INDIFFERENCE	Clary sage
	Jasmine (absolute)
	Patchouli
	Rose (absolute)
	Sandlewood
	Ylang-ylang
STRESS, NERVOUS TENSION	Bergamot*
	Chamomile
	Frankincense
	Myrrh
	Rose (absolute)
	Sandlewood

*When wearing full-strength bergamot, be careful not to expose your skin to intense sunlight or ultraviolet light as skin discoloration may result.

Aromatherapy Formulas for Reducing Depression

Essential oils work synergistically—that is, they complement and enhance one another's properties when mixed. For this reason, it is usually best to blend between two and four oils with the desired properties and with aromas pleasing to the user. Mixing more than four together will tend to reduce the strength of the mixture.

Many scents can reduce depression or symptoms related to depression. The scent of jasmine, for example, stimulates changes in the front of the brain, causing us to be more alert. The scent of lavender affects the back of the brain, producing a more relaxed state. Consequently, sufferers of insomnia may benefit from a few drops of lavender on their pillow to induce a more restful sleep. A sniff of jasmine in the morning can be a substitute for caffeine.

The following aromatherapy combinations should be used four times daily:

- For short-term mild depression, combine four parts ylang-ylang, four parts clary sage, three parts geranium, two parts basil, and one part sandalwood. Use four times daily.
- For chronic depression, combine equal parts of basil, clary sage, jasmine, rose, and German chamomile (*Matricaria recutita*).
- For manic behavior, combine equal parts of geranium, lavender, neroli, and sandalwood.
- For general depression, combine equal parts of bergamot, lavender, neroli, and basil.

Always store essential oils, either alone or in combination, in dark glass bottles.

Some food oils have been tested successfully for mood disorders. They include green apple and cucumber for claustrophobia, and vanilla, nutmeg, and apple for various forms of anxiety. In meditation, visualization, or hypnosis, vanilla oil can help individuals recall childhood memories that might help them to move beyond their depression.

Aside from reducing the appetite, food aromas have also been found useful in relieving frustration. Because a pleasant odor can remind a person of a childhood memory of happy times, scents reduce frustration. So food aromas can help you reduce depression related to body image and weight, because they reduce the frustration that leads to cravings.

Ways to Employ Essential Oils

Most people who include essential oils as part of their daily regime have one or two favorite methods for employing them. The four most popular are bathing, inhalation, massage, and room dispersal.

Bathing

Bathing, when used for more than personal cleanliness, can actually be called water balancing. Bathing with aromatic oils can help correct or prevent emotional and structural imbalances and maintain or improve overall well-being. The use of water as a balancing and healing tool can help maintain good health by increasing the elimination of metabolic wastes and improving blood and lymphatic circulation. Herbal baths and special showers can increase the activity of internal organs as well as of the largest organ of all, the skin. If you have low energy, water balancing can give you a boost, and if you are overstimulated, water can soothe and sedate you. When combined with massage and other hands-on healing techniques, water balancing with herbal oils is very beneficial in dealing with mood disorders.

To heal depression, work up to taking an aromatherapy bath three times a week. Two good aromatherapy formulas to use are:

- For general stress, five to six drops each of chamomile, hyssop, lavendar, marjoram, chamomile, and rosemary. This formula will stimulate the skin; relax tense, sore muscles; and relieve headaches, fatigue, and nervous tension.
- For mild depression, three drops lavender, three drops ylang-ylang, two drops basil, two drops geranium, and one drop grapefruit.

Fill the bathtub with warm water and add your chosen oil combination as well as a tablespoon of sweet almond oil. Stir the water well using your hands, then sit in the bath for twenty to thirty minutes.

Inhalation

Uncorking the bottle and taking a big sniff is not the way to inhale the scent of an essential oil. Instead, the proper way is to sprinkle six to eight drops of essence on a tissue and inhale deeply three times. Another method is to add three to four drops to a basin of hot water. Close your eyes, lean over the basin with a towel over your head to trap the vapors, and inhale deeply several times. A good formula to use is equal parts of benzoin, eucalyptus, pine, and spruce, which will also relieve the sinus congestion resulting from a common cold. *Caution*: Do not try this method if you have asthma. Note also that concentrated steam can cause choking.

A third way to inhale the scent of an essential oil is to place one to two drops on the edge of your pillow.

Massage

One of the most popular ways to use aromatherapy oils is in massage. The fastest way to get the oils into your system is by mixing the essence with a carrier oil, then rubbing the compound on your chest morning and night. Oils such as coriander, vertivert, cinnamon, ylang-ylang, and neroli are a few of many that work to improve circulation and relax the nervous system.

A good formula for a concentrated massage oil for mild depression is two teaspoons sweet almond oil (the carrier oil), eight drops ylang-ylang, eight drops lavender, two drops geranium, two drops basil, and two drops bergamot. Apply a small amount of this oil combination on the backs of the hands, on the chest area, or around the navel, and inhale deeply.

The carrier oil acts as a lubricating base and protects the skin from the potent essential oils. Carrier oils must be of vegetable origin and fine textured, with little or no smell. Apricot kernel, almond, canola, evening primrose, grapeseed, safflower, and sunflower oils are all good. Other popular carrier oils are avocado, olive, and wheat germ. These last are much thicker, which is good for dry skin, and are usually mixed with a lighter carrier oil such as grapeseed. In general, the correct ratio of essence to carrier oil is six drops to two teaspoons.

Once combined, store the massage oil in a labeled dark glass bottle.

Room Dispersal

An essence can be effectively dispersed throughout a room by use of an atomizer. Another good method is to buy a small heat lamp with a crucible. The heat vaporizes the essence and disperses it throughout the room. Heat lamps are available at many stores that sell essences.

Nebulizers mist microscopic essential oil droplets into the air quickly.

You can also purchase aromalamps, aromatherapy candles, and incense.

Whichever method you choose, the proper way to breathe in the essence is as follows:

1. Stand with your feet six inches apart. Clasp your fingers together in front of you and let your arms relax.
2. Inhale deeply while you bring your clasped hands straight over your head. (As the arms move up on the inhalation, imagine them floating on the breath.) Let your forearms fall behind your head.
3. Pause and hold your breath to the count of three.
4. Place a little pressure on the heels of your hands, and start your exhalation as your arms return to where they began in front of you. Exhale the aroma slowly.
5. Repeat this cycle for a total of ten inhalations and exhalations.

Don't use aromatic blends every day or diffuse them for long periods of time as your sense of smell will begin to "ignore" the aroma, thereby, reducing the therapeutic effects.

Some Cautions

Essential oils, like all plant products, should always be stored in tightly closed, dark glass bottles to prevent deterioration. In addition, like the plants they come from, they may be dangerous if used over an extended period of time. It is strongly recommended that you limit yourself to the external methods unless someone is supervising you with experience in internal applications. If the condition being treated does not show measurable improvement after a few days of application, consult a trained medical practitioner who has access to sophisticated diagnostic techniques.

With any powerful healing agent, it is possible that an individual may demonstrate a hypersensitivity to a particular oil. It is, therefore, important to test the oil in question on a patch of skin in a sensitive area before full-scale use. As valuable as these oils are, it is important to remember that aromatic oils may be contraindicated if you suffer from asthma or migraine headaches, or experience shortness of breath or eye irritation when using them.[3]

7   BALANCING THE EMOTIONS WITH FLOWER REMEDIES

There is no one reason for depression. Each depressed individual will have a unique history of dysfunctional relationships, traumatic childhood, stress, financial hardships, insomnia and sleep disorders, unresolved grief, genetic predisposition, aging, serious physical illness, or family environment. Individually or in combination, some or all of these factors may initiate a downward spiraling cycle that results in depression. Herbal-based flower remedies help to heal depression on a vibrational-energetic level. These homeopathically prepared plant essences support the depressed individual in recognizing and addressing issues such as personal growth, self-observation, forgiveness, getting in touch with repressed feelings, expressing gratitude, effective communication, ending procrastination, making choices instead of excuses, ending self-isolation, impatience, hopelessness, a sense of impending doom, and despondency.

In this chapter, we will examine flower remedies—what they are, how they work, and how to use them. We'll also take a look at the man who first developed them, Dr. Edward Bach.

The Emotions, Flower Remedies, and Energetic Imbalances

General emotional stress, trauma, spiritual longing, and energetic imbalances alone or in combination are all major causes of depression. In the case of situational depression, the ability of a person to control responses to stress, rather than becoming a victim of unpleasant situations, has a great impact on the healing process. Homeopathy is one system for doing this. There are many different systems of energetically based flower remedies; however, by far the most commonly used and most easily available are those developed in the 1930s by the British pathologist, homeopath, and research scientist (in bacteriology, pathology, and immunology) Dr. Edward Bach. Dr. Bach took the vibrational principles so frequently associated with Chinese and Ayurvedic medicine today and applied them to balancing emotional states through homeopathically prepared flower remedies. Bach discovered that behind every patient's situational depression and emotional and psychological disturbances is a vibrational link.

Over a number of years, Dr. Bach isolated remedies, one by one. Each remedy was intended to treat a different negative and counterproductive emotion. He discovered that picking certain species of wildflowers at certain times in their blooming cycle and preparing them homeopathically maximized their vibrationally based healing qualities. Eliminating toxic plants or those that might produce side effects, he discovered thirty-eight flowering plants, trees, and special waters that had profound influence on balancing various dysfunctional behavior patterns as well as different mental and emotional stresses.

By looking beyond the limitations of allopathic medicine and the psychoanalytic approach dominant at that time, he was able to take into account the feelings of his patients rather than just treating their psychological symptoms. By addressing the cause-and-effect relationship of pain when dealing with illness, he bridged the gap between physical and emotional pain.

Bach was able to see before virtually any Western physicians or researchers the strong link between emotional imbalance and immunity. He describes in his writings that emotional challenges, especially loss of hope, worry, anxiety, resentment, feelings of despair, fear, and a lack of self-confidence, can deplete a patient's vitality to the extent that he or she may lose natural resistance and become susceptible to a host of physical illnesses.

Today one would be hard-pressed to find a knowledgeable, progressive-thinking scientist or physician who does not at least look into the psychological and emotional variables affecting an individual when attempting to treat a physical illness.

Dr. Bach's remedies were and still are prepared by placing the petals and blooms of the specific herb in spring water and allowing sunlight to activate their potential. This process is a homeopathic approach called *potentising* of the remedy. This sun-"energized" liquid is then naturally preserved with a small amount of brandy. Those who wish to avoid all al-cohol can place the liquid in very hot water to evaporate the brandy.

Because they are "energetically based," the Bach Flower Remedies offer a spiritual dimension to the healing of depression. The remedies create a system for bolstering faith and hope. Dr. Bach's system is based on the concept that everyone deserves love and that there is a power greater than ourselves that will help us to restore love and sanity in our lives. The flower remedies are not a crutch; they are a vehicle for clarity.

In fact, if you accidentally choose a remedy that is inappropriate for a specific emotional state, the remedy will have no effect at all, remaining neutral. The remedies do not work biochemically but rather by gently reestablishing emotional and psychological equilibrium through ener-getic, or vibrational, shifts. While other drug-based approaches as well as many herbs and nutrients address brain chemistry and depression, the flower remedies do not specifically influence brain chemistry nor do they target specific symptoms. Rather, they address the state of mind of the depressed or emotionally stressed individual. They balance chi by going to the person's energy source. These remedies are considered a transfor-mation event in the treatment of emotional problems through natural healing and homeopathy.

These flower remedies have been used for over fifty years by medical doctors and psychologists, as well as the general public. Many mental health professionals integrate these gentle homeopathic remedies into an emotional healing program specifically for depression. They are available in most natural-food stores and are easily prepared by adding a few drops to spring water.

The Flower Remedies and Depression

All thirty-eight flower remedies may affect depression in some indi-rect way, and therefore, I will discuss them all and describe how they can help alleviate a depressed state. They are listed alphabetically in this chap-ter. I had the opportunity to study in 1976 at Mount Vernon, Dr. Bach's home in England, and later with Marjorie Spaulding, a long-term master of the remedies who had herself studied with Nora Weeks, Dr. Bach's successor. I also developed a long and deep friendship with the late Leslie Kaslof, who through his family's Elon distributing company, had a major role in gaining recognition for the remedies in the American healing community. A master herbalist, Leslie pointed out that the remedies that seemed to be most specific for depression were gorse, gentian, mustard, and sweet chestnut. Through my own experience, I have seen these four remedies, particularly gorse, help depressed individuals who consistently experienced feelings of hopelessness and despair.

Rescue Remedy, a special flower remedy formula, may be of great help at times of extreme trauma. It is a combination of five Bach remedies and is used in situational depression where there has been a sudden trauma, an anxiety attack, or a general crisis.

In subtle ways, flower remedies can assist a person in reducing patterns that feed depression. This may be done without necessarily addressing the underlying cause of fear and anxiety. I have personally found this technique to be effective when combined with a variation of an approach known as systemic desensitization. This is a stress-reducing technique in which a client is taught to visualize an enlivening mental image and focus on this image throughout the day.

All of the flower remedies influence the emotions on some level and most affect depression whether it is connected to despair, fear, or some other emotion. Changing is seldom easy. You may feel that you can't go forward, and yet you are fearful of remaining in the same place. You feel as if you are stuck between a rock and a hard place. This dilemma can create a sense of hopelessness and loss of faith. You fear that you may never break out of this cycle, and that you may sink into deeper despair and depression.

The Bach Flower Remedies offer a way out of negative self-talk, helping you to be honest about the reality of your life and helping you to:

- Strengthen your focus on positive life choices even when you are depressed.
- Be honest with yourself about what situations make you glad, mad, depressed, sad, or so on.
- Address your emotional needs in healthy ways.
- Express your feelings.

If you are depressed, even if there is no definable reason, these remedies can guide you to feeling more emotionally balanced and support you in recognizing and addressing issues such as personal growth, ending procrastination, forgiving, getting in touch with repressed feelings, expressing gratitude, hopelessness, effective communication, self-observation, making choices instead of excuses, ending self-isolation, impatience, despondency, and a sense of impending doom.

Once you become familiar with the different remedies, you can prepare combinations that fit your specific needs.

Using the Flower Remedies

Using the flower remedies is not difficult. The following directions are based on the system used at the Bach Center in England, where Dr. Bach lived and practiced.

Pick the remedy or remedies you are going to use and place two drops in a small glass of spring water (not distilled or filtered water) and sip at intervals throughout the day or until relief is obtained. Replenish as necessary. For longer-term use, add two drops to a 30-milliliter dropper bottle and take four drops from this solution four times daily or more frequently if necessary, until relief is obtained. If you feel that they address a wide range of emotional patterns, then up to six or seven remedies may be taken together if required. In the beginning, however, try to keep it simple.

Change the remedies to adjust to mood changes. You cannot overdose or hurt yourself from long-term use of the Bach Flower Remedies, and there is no limit to how long you can take your chosen remedy or remedies.

The Flower Remedies

Following are the Bach Flower Remedies and how they relate to situational and trauma-based depression.

Agrimony

Agrimony is helpful for those who feel unloved but who present a cheery disposition in order to hide their pain from others. They sometimes exhibit manic behavior and are also fearful that if others know their internal pain, they may become a burden to them. Agrimony types may drink or be prone to drug use to escape from their unexpressed emotional pain.

Aspen

Aspen is valuable for overanxious individuals who are fearful and apprehensive without clear cause. Aspen dispels stress, and aids in relaxation.

Beech

Beech is the remedy for those who are self-critical to a fault. These individuals may also be perfectionists who tend to find fault in just about everything and everyone. They are critical and inclined to overreact to small idiosyncrasies or annoyances in others. Beech helps these people to see that there is great benefit in choosing opportunities that present a reduced opportunity for failure or disappointment.

Centaury

Centaury is the remedy for introverts who are overeager to please others, even if their own needs are being ignored or left for later. Often making resolutions and commitments that they seem to be unable to keep, they are easily dominated and exploited. This creates a sense of emptiness that leads to depression. No matter what they do, they experience a sense of dissatisfaction that will continue to grow as they ignore their real needs. In an attempt to compensate for their neediness, they aim to please others, but their aim is off center. Centaury helps target a person's needs, and supports him or her in acting on these needs.

Cerato

Cerato is valuable for individuals who make poor decisions and lack confidence in their own judgments. These individuals are constantly seeking guidance from others without considering the quality of the advice. They often leave open the possibility for bad advice. Their lack of confidence creates an environment that can lead to depression.

Cherry Plum

Cherry plum is valuable for the fear of losing mental and physical control or of doing something desperate. People who experience this type of fear may have impulses to do things known or thought to be wrong and become depressed in response to this impulse.

Chestnut Bud

Chestnut bud is recommended for those who repeat the same destructive pattern again and again. They fail to learn from their mistakes and past experience.

Chicory

Chicory is valuable for people who experience the need to control or direct those close to them. The need to control can lead to frustration when they are unable to fulfill this need.

Clematis

Clematis is for individuals who seem out of touch with reality. They are often late and inconsistent with commitments they make with others. They have little concern for the present and live with their heads in the clouds.

Crab Apple

Crab apple is useful for individuals who suffer from low self-esteem and have an obsessive-compulsive attitude concerning cleanliness. They are fearful of being contaminated and allow this compulsion to dominate their life.

Elm

Elm helps to ease painful feelings of inadequacy and of being overwhelmed with responsibility—feelings that can leave a sense that there is no escape from the pressures of life. This can elevate until the person becomes depressed.

Gentian

Gentian helps an individual to build confidence by alleviating self-doubt and discouragement. To transcend depression, it is important for a person to have hope for success in the future and not get easily discouraged.

If you suffer from a chronic disease, gentian and gorse make the best combination. For resignation and apathy, gentian and wild rose make an effective combination.

Gorse

Gorse is for feelings of hopelessness and futility. A person in this state may abuse drugs or alcohol. Gorse helps these individuals to retain hope and remember that there is a light at the end of the tunnel.

If you suffer from a chronic disease, gorse and gentian are the best combination.

Heather

Heather is helpful for those who seek companionship from anyone who will listen to their problems and for those who have difficulty being alone. It helps people to be more comfortable with themselves and helps them to be more selective in whom they seek companionship from.

Holly

Holly is for those who experience feelings of envy, jealousy, suspicion, and revenge out of the need for love, a feeling that can also lead to possessiveness and depression. For anger and frustration, holly and vervain make an effective combination.

Honeysuckle

Honeysuckle helps those weighed down by regret and attachments to the past. Sometimes a person who is depressed will reminisce about a time in the past when things were better rather than focusing on creating contentment in the present.

Hornbeam

Hornbeam helps depressed individuals address feelings of being fatigued. It diminishes the sense that one is unable to face the day—and other feelings that create laziness, a lack of energy, and a deeper sense of depression.

Impatiens

Impatiens relieves impatience and diminishes the sense that every moment must be acted on quickly and that everyone else is moving too slowly. This type of impatience often leads to frustration and depression.

Larch

Larch boosts confidence and reduces or eliminates the fear of failure that often causes people to slip from a balanced functional life into deep depression.

Mimulus

Mimulus is valuable for those suffering from unreasonable phobias and fears of, for example, spiders, snakes, the dark, and heights. A phobia may appear as an eating disorder such as anorexia or bulemia.

Mustard

Mustard brings clarity and relief from depression and emotional darkness of unexplained onset.

Oak

Oak helps a person maintain balance and consistency in personal healthcare. This is valuable for those individuals inclined to get involved in extreme or unbalanced health fads.

Olive

Olive is best used for mental and physical exhaustion, and sapped vitality with no reserve. This is the type of overwhelming personal ordeal that can bring on depression.

Pine

Pine reduces the tendency to be hard on oneself to the extent of taking the blame for another's mistakes. The anxiety created by this kind of behavior can lead to frustration and depression.

Red Chestnut

Red chestnut reduces the type of situational depression that results from worry over the hardships or misfortunes of loved ones.

Rock Rose

Rock rose is helpful in reducing feelings of panic, terror, or nightmares. Individuals who suffer in this way may use food, alcohol, or other drugs to find a sense of safety as well as the peace, comfort, and emotional nourishment they are lacking. For these individuals, this self-destructive behavior becomes a sort of security blanket.

Rock Water

Rock water is valuable for those of rigid, almost inflexible, personality and style. These individuals like strict guidelines in everyday life and have an intense desire to maintain an ideal, fulfill a goal, or set an example even to the point of diminishing return.

Scleranthus

Scleranthus is valuable for those who have difficulty making decisions, including positive choices about day-to-day lifestyle patterns. This is the remedy if you eat poorly or have irregular exercise patterns. When you are already in the depths of depression and are looking for an easy way out of the darkness, scleranthus can help you move in the right direction. Scleranthus is the remedy of choice during PMS-based depression.

Star of Bethlehem

Star of Bethlehem helps to pacify the state of grief or trauma caused by a great personal loss. This remedy is valuable for those suffering from culturally specific depression.

Sweet Chestnut

Sweet chestnut helps ease feelings of despair and absolute bleakness that give you a sense that life is overwhelming or that you can't go on. Such feelings often lead to depression.

Vervain

Vervain is useful for those who are argumentative and always want to have the last word. They frequently believe that no one is listening to them. This reaction is often a compensation that comes from childhood experiences of being told to keep quiet. This "oral" frustration can result in depression. This remedy works especially together with dance and movement therapy.

Vine

Vine is for individuals who are natural leaders. They have a need to be in charge, and when in balance, they are very empowering to others. When emotionally out of balance, these individuals can become obsessively controlling, even dictatorial. Feelings of insecurity lead to this type of aggression.

Walnut

Walnut helps with sudden or extreme emotional transitions. These are often associated with hormonal changes such as during puberty or menopause. It is also the remedy most appropriate for bipolar disorder.

Water Violet

Water violet is helpful for loners and those who prefer to bear emotional burdens on their own. These individuals seldom seek the support of others and believe that they must be self-reliant at all costs. Even if they find themselves deeply depressed, they will turn down support, group therapy work, or twelve-step-style meetings where they can remain anonymous. This pattern can lead to the social isolation that may result in even deeper depression.

White Chestnut

White chestnut is helpful for manic personalities, especially those individuals with fast-moving, cluttered minds whose lives are so filled with constant chatter and diversions that concentration or focus on any one thing becomes virtually impossible.

Wild Oat

Wild oat is appropriate for those who desire more from life but have lost hope that there are any options available. They are often in careers where they work just hard enough to keep from being fired and are paid just enough to keep them from quitting. They are dissatisfied with their current situation in life and often feel as if they have not or cannot attain a goal they've set for themselves. Being discouraged with life or oneself can create the frustration that leads to depression.

Wild Rose

Wild rose is a great remedy for those committed to making a new start. It is especially appropriate since a new program always involves a change and wild rose aids those with a desire to change their lives but who have resigned themselves to their current position. For resignation and apathy, gentian and wild rose make an effective combination.

Willow

Willow is for anger and regrets concerning the past. This flower helps reduce feelings of bitterness and resentment, often related to feeling as though one has been treated unfairly or dealt a bad hand in life. Such feelings can lead to depression.

Flower Remedy Combinations

Here are a few additional combinations of flower remedies and the specific situations related to depression for which I have seen them work effectively:

- Obsessive-compulsive disorder—crab apple, heather, and white chestnut
- Fatigue exhaustion—olive and hornbeam
- Fear—aspen, cherry plum, mimulus, red chestnut, and rock rose
- Insomnia—white chestnut, olive, and vervain
- Emotional insecurity and lack of confidence—larch, centaury, and cerato
- Loneliness—water violet and heather
- Stress—olive, vervain, elm, and oak
- Suicidal thoughts—cherry plum and agrimony
- Worry—white chestnut, agrimony, and red chestnut
- Situation depression—walnut, larch, mimulus, aspen, and scleranthus

Buying Flower Remedies

Bach Flower Remedies are available in 10-milliliter (1/3 ounce) bottles. They can be found at many natural-food and health-food markets. If you have difficulty obtaining them, see "Resources" on page 233.

8 ❧ THE BODY-MIND-SPIRIT APPROACH TO HEALING DEPRESSION

A large-scale Harvard Medical School study, published in the *New England Journal of Medicine*, found that depression was among the top five conditions for which people were more likely to seek alternative treatments—with or without mainstream treatment approaches. Among the most popular of those alternative treatments are those that integrate the health of not just the body, but the mind and spirit as well.

The Body-Mind Connection

Psychologists know that the mind ascends quickly to what it believes to be the truth. It grabs at any declaration, proposition, or alleged fact. It creates evidence to support its beliefs, even if there is no personal knowledge to support it. In addition, many of those beliefs are based on unresolved memories that may or may not be available to the conscious mind.

Stop whatever you are doing for just a few minutes. Now pay attention to the inner working of your mind. Do you see how it keeps switching from one thought to another? It is almost impossible to focus the mind. It's as if it is incapable of stopping at any one idea. Instead, it wanders from this to that, and from that to something else. The mind is like a television screen with thousands of images coming and going. At the same time that you are watching the television screen, there are millions of other images on the other channels. We stay with one channel for a while, get bored, and switch to the next channel. I call this "mental channel surfing." Rather than being strange or unusual, this is the ordinary state of our mind. Many educators complain that students have shorter attention spans now than ten or fifteen years ago. However, this is the ongoing state of the mind—our individual personality bouncing from one sense to another, one thought to another, like a butterfly going from one leaf to another.

The more someone desires something, the more he or she focuses attention upon it, and in turn, the more this desire grows. The longer someone desires, the greater the desire becomes. The greater the desire is, the more difficult it is to abstain from this thing. The desire may even become all-consuming.

Desire is nothing more than repeated mental imagery that has become a habit, sometimes with an emotional component and an associated physical action or habit. It is nothing more than forms made up of textures, sounds, tastes, colors, and aromas. Sometimes these desires lead to destructive patterns, fears, and depression. The delusion toward, and illusion of, these things drag humankind away from our true destiny—a simple, joyous life.

Instead, we are often dragged toward destruction. At one point in time, a person may sincerely believe he or she knows something about something, only to realize later that the information was completely inaccurate. Likewise, another person may have great knowledge about something and not even be aware that he or she possesses such knowledge.

As Chinese philosopher Chuang Tsu said:

> Whether or not I am able to define what the true nature of this soul is, it is irrelevant to the soul itself. The soul enters a physical body, which runs its course until it is exhausted. The struggle and abrasions of life harass it, and it is driven relentlessly on this path without possibility of slowing the process. Is this not a pitiful state? To be worn out by life without living to enjoy the fruit of this labor, and then to die without even knowing when this event will come to pass. Is not this a just cause for grief?[1]

In recent years, the view of human behavior has been modified as developing technologies reveal the brain's workings in increasing detail. The mind is a complex thing. Psychoneuroimmunologists now tell us that, scientifically, body and brain are one and the same with the function or dysfunction of one instantly affecting the other. Psychoneuroimmunology research has produced evidence that our thought patterns specifically, and instantaneously, affect our body chemistry and can even suppress our immune system.

Every day scientists are surprised at the workings of the human mind. What seemed mysterious one day may be obvious the next, and then some new piece of information arises to make it all mysterious again. For instance, various studies conducted in recent years indicate that, in the short term at least, placebos can be as effective as antidepressants.

The Subconscious Mind

The subconscious mind is able to contradict the laws of logic in a way that the conscious mind cannot. The laws of logic, no matter how objective they attempt to be, are still about the subjective, for thought is subjective and logic comes from thought. In the mind, everything is theoretical and reality is simply a special case of the theoretical. Our common reality makes perfect intellectual sense if not looked at too closely, but in time, we soon learn that it is impossible to live with any intellectual concept of reality when so many contradictions arise. It is these contradictions that can lead a deeply intellectual, rational mind to depression.

Connecting to the subconscious mind does not come through intellectual understanding. It is only by detaching from the illusion created through the conscious senses that one can create a new reality in the mind. This realization does not come about through wishing it so. It comes from applying the natural qualities of the mind in a new direction. Many body-mind researchers take the position that a person's natural suggestibility, when combined with hopes and beliefs concerning their treatment, might cause a significant shift in their biochemistry, which of course would then influence the individual's physiology and emotional state. In essence, suggestibility may have an important role to play in the healing of depression, especially in the impact it may have on the placedo effect.

Intuition

One of the strongest elements of body-mind healing is an expansion of intuitive sensibilities. As you continue to practice inner inquiry, you will find that you are developing sensitivity to what intuition communicates, and you trust these messages more and more. More often than not, this "intuitive information" doesn't come in verbal or logical form. In fact, in the beginning, you are not even aware that you are developing this level of intuitive sensitivity.

Intuition may show up for each of us differently but researchers find that it is generally experienced in three specific ways:

- Physical sensations. Kinesthetic intuitives experience physical sensations that communicate information. They will physically feel "comfortable" or "uncomfortable" about something. This may appear as a gut feeling, a physical pain, or something that excites their heart.
- Emotional intuition. This is usually experienced as a vague or specific feeling that has no explanation, but is usually right. You might feel slightly depressed because you know something is wrong. You actually become sensitive to the emotional states of others around you. You see their posture or you automatically have a feeling arise when they say something. It is not intellectual. It happens right there in that moment. Emotional intuitives often say words such as, "I like" and "I don't like," or "This feels good [or bad] to me." They respond to requests from others and make decisions based on how they feel. If they are not conscious of this quality, they may experience a feeling without realizing that they are picking up thoughts and feelings from another person.
- Mental intuition. Mental intuition can resemble a thought. It may simply be an internal conversation you are having with yourself about a solution to a problem. It could be a brainstorm in the shower, a hunch, or a nagging thought that won't go away in the mind of a person who is not normally obsessive about thoughts. Mental intuition is not logical but you might initially experience it as if it is. These thoughts are about common sense and what seems obvious. It is a more goal-oriented sensibility than the other two forms of intuition.

"Most often people have a combination of the above three, though one form may be dominant," says Nancy Rosanoff, a respected writer and speaker on intuition. "Rarely is someone totally one type. We categorize them only to indicate that there is more than one way to perceive intuitive information."[2]

The Placebo Effect

A *placebo* (Latin for "I shall please") is a treatment—most often a medication—believed by the administrator of the treatment to be innocuous or inert. Researchers and medical doctors sometimes give placebos such as sugar or starch pills to groups of patients (a control group) for the purpose of determining whether a drug being given to another group has any more medicinal value than the placebo itself. Placebos are not limited to pills, however. "Fake psychotherapy" and "fake surgery" are also used as placebos.

The current interest in the placebo effect was most probably ignited over a hundred years ago by H. K. Beecher who, while evaluating over two dozen studies, calculated that 30 percent of those in the studies improved owing to the placebo effect. Some studies calculate the placebo effect as being even greater than what Beecher claimed. For example, some studies have shown that placebos are effective in 50 or 60 percent of subjects with certain conditions, including depression, and may be as effective as some of the new psychotropic drugs used in the treatment of various brain disorders. However, there is not even enough evidence from studies at this time to prove that these drugs are more effective than placebos.

The process of how the placebo effect functions might be through the following sequence of events:

1. Much of our behavior and many of our beliefs are learned.
2. Sensory experiences and beliefs can affect neurochemistry.
3. The body's neurochemical system influences, and is influenced by, other biochemical systems, including the immune and hormonal systems.
4. These systems can affect physiological and emotional health, particularly depression.

Attitude

Current scientific knowledge supports the idea that a person's positive or hopeful attitude and beliefs may be key to their physical and emotional well-being and recovery from illness and injury. Part of a "sick" person's behavior is learned. Since many behaviors are the role-play of a person within certain culturally and socially based belief systems, cultural factors can also bring a placebo effect into play. Role-playing is not synonymous with faking a cure since the person faking a cure will be shown, through various diagnostic and measuring procedures, to still have the specific affliction. Any changes brought about through the placebo effect can be measured, by changes in how one acts and how one feels, as well as by shifts in attitude and alterations in body chemistry.

This brings us to the power of suggestion as a therapeutic tool. All people respond to suggestions. Mentally and emotionally, healthy people respond to positive suggestions. However, all people, whether or not they are emotionally healthy, are not all suggestible in the same way. In a study of asthmatic patients, scientists found that they could produce dilation of the airways by telling people they were inhaling a bronchodilator. Research has also shown that the power of suggestion, when offered to a person in a particular psychological state with certain belief systems, and offered in a certain tone with certain words, can help reduce or eliminate pain.

Based on what is known about the mind and how it may respond to certain suggestions, research indicates that the most effective therapeutic program should include constant attention from the patient's support system. This includes caring, affection, encouragement, supporting a sense of hope, healing touch, and other positive interpersonal support, combined with stress-reduction tools. This, and a reduction in uncertainty about what treatment to take or what the outcome will be, may assist in the release of endorphins and other positive body chemicals. These factors, when combined with an effective therapist and attention to biochemical causative factors, may trigger physical and psychological reactions that promote healing.

Studies indicate that just being in a healing environment or circumstance may have an effect. According to a *New York Times* article, "Depressed patients who are merely put on a waiting list for treatment do not do as well as those given placebos."[3]

The Brain Wave Factor

It is now known that how we think, what we think about, and how connected we are to the subconscious aspect of our mind can be measured by evaluating what level of brain waves are dominant at any particular time. In fact, throughout the day we have constant shifts in our brain wave patterns. Certain activities and processes—including emotional changes in the brain—produce measurable brain wave activity. Brain waves can be measured (as cycles per second, called hertz), and an understanding of brain waves can be an important tool in addressing mental and emotional health issues. The four primary distinct varieties of brain waves are:

- Beta waves (14 to 100 hertz). These are the most rapid of the brain waves and are active when you are in a normal waking state. This pattern is associated with concentration, alertness, cognition, arousal, and very elevated anxiety levels.
- Alpha waves (8 to 13 hertz). These waves are dominant when you are daydreaming or feeling calm and tranquil or mentally unfocused. Light music, many types of classical music, and any external influences that seem to reduce stress are generally connected to the alpha state. Healthy individuals who have consistently low levels of stress tend to produce an abundance of alpha activity. Meditation, creative visualization, as well as imagining, occur in alpha.
- Theta waves (4 to 8 hertz). This is the brain wave pattern associated with the twilight state between waking and sleep. It is a slower, more powerfully rhythmic pattern that is commonly accompanied by unexpected, dreamlike images.
- Delta waves (below 4 hertz). When you are asleep or unconscious, your brain waves are in delta. It is in this state that your brain is stimulated to manufacture essential brain chemicals such as serotonin, and release large quantities of healing growth hormones.

The process of guiding someone into alpha or theta states is known as induction. This can take place through music and color therapy, or through visualization, meditation, or hypnosis. Hypnosis, meditation, and visualization will not always be effective tools in working with depression. People who are highly suggestible may not easily go into alpha or theta states. Conversely, those individuals who easily go into alpha and theta states may not be highly suggestible.

However, those individuals who are highly suggestible and who enter more easily into alpha and theta are more suggestible when in these states. This is wonderful news for the depressed person since a guided process into alpha or theta can help them to become free of this depression. There is no magic to it. Induction is something you can do with a specially trained individual, or it is a process you can be taught to do and can practice on your own. The more you practice, the better you get at it.

Suggestibility and Memory

How suggestible we are or are not is influenced by how events that have taken place in our life are recorded by the subconscious mind. Some memories are unresolved. These memories belong to one of two distinct categories. The first category is composed of disturbing, haunting, never-leaving painful memories that prevent a person from being present in the moment. Always thinking of the past or the future, these people are often highly dysfunctional. Depression based on post-traumatic stress disorder belongs in this category. Traumatic circumstances that have taken place in late childhood or in young adulthood may also cause this condition.

The second category is composed of suppressed memories. A suppressed memory is a memory that is contained in the subconscious mind. This is a state that most of us exist in. In fact, we are usually unaware of many details of traumatic experiences we have had, and of the emotional impact they had—and continue to have—on us. Individuals with suppressed memories are generally functional in life but have specific areas of dysfunction. The popular culture term used to describe the source of these specific dysfunctions is "emotional baggage"—the emotional luggage of life that you carry around with you wherever you go that influences most of your relationships.

Consciousness Shifting

A suggestibility script is a system of structured steps used to encourage and reinforce suggestions. A script can be used in meditation, visualization, or when working with a professional hypnotist, pastoral counselor, or therapist. Scripts are designed to bring a person, who gives permission, into an alpha or theta trance state, where new internalized thought processes (anchors) can be placed to shift from reactive to proactive behavior. All behavior, after all, is consciously or unconsciously controlled by reinforcement and encouragement. This positive reinforcement results in a shift of consciousness and of attitude. The sequence of consciousness shifting in alpha or theta is as follows:

1. Suggestions are made when the client is open to a positive shift in habit. These suggestions are reinforced through visual, auditory, or

kinesthetic anchors. (Reinforcement is any action or thing that strengthens a habit.) Many people receive negative reinforcement from their friends or surrounding environment. This can be counterproductive.

2. We all need to believe in something, and these positive suggestions given while in alpha or theta create a shift in belief (remember, a belief is something you hold to be true even though there may be no physical or logical evidence to support the belief).

3. With a shift in belief, there is an emotional shift.

4. With the shift in emotions and feelings, there is an attitudinal change.

5. The shift in attitude creates a shift in behavior and a resultant experience of life.

6. The shift in experience brings the successful achievement of stated goals and the passing of depression.

Through each of these steps, there is positive reinforcement and encouragement.

Consciousness-Shifting Scripts

The following scripts can be used as an opening sequence before any meditation, visualization process, or other alpha- or theta-inducing process. Remember, when you visualize an activity, your muscles respond to electrical impulses just as they would when you are actually engaged in the same activity you are imagining. This is a mental and emotional exercise session. When you do this, it is best to create very vivid images and, if possible, bring all of your senses into play. If it is a "nature" visualization, smell the aromas and hear the sounds of the forest in your mind as if you were actually there.

Visualization for Manic Behavior

This visualization is designed to remove you from what is known in Asia as the "Monkey Mind"—the fast, jumping around of thoughts that is common in manic behavior.

Record the following on a cassette or compact disc using a slow, calm voice. To use the recording, lie down flat on your back with your eyes closed.

Beginning at your toes and working up toward your head, feel each section of your body totally relax. Feet. Ankles. Lower legs. Knees. Thighs. Buttocks. Abdomen. Lower back. Chest. Upper back. Shoulders. Upper arms. Forearms. Hands. Wrists. Neck. Jaw. Eyes. Eyebrows. Scalp. Observe your breathing process and stay aware of your breaths. Inhale. Exhale. Inhale. Exhale.

Self-Induction to Replace Depressive Thoughts

Record the following on a cassette or compact disc using a slow, calm voice. To use the recording, sit or lie in a comfortable position with your eyes closed.

Imagine yourself in a place you like very much . . . by a lake, or on the ocean. Perhaps you are floating gently on a sailboat on a peaceful lake on a warm, summer day.

You are continuing to relax even more now. And you continue becoming more comfortable. This is your own world, which you like very much. You are going to find that anytime you want to spend a few minutes by yourself relaxing and feeling very comfortable and serene, you can automatically go back to this feeling you're experiencing now. You can put yourself into this world anytime you like.

There are specific times when you will want to feel this serene feeling. Remember, it is yours whenever you want.

Continue enjoying this pleasant experience as your subconscious mind is receiving everything I tell you. You will be pleased with the way you automatically respond to everything.

Self-Induction for Rational or Intellectual Individuals

Record the following on a cassette or compact disc using a slow, calm voice. To use the recording, sit or lie in a comfortable position with your eyes closed.

Breathe steadily and evenly, just as though you were pretending to be sound asleep. Breathe so evenly, so steadily, that you almost wouldn't disturb a feather placed immediately in front of you. The feather doesn't move.

As you allow yourself to relax even more, see if you can sense the beating of your own heart. Once you have sensed the rhythm of your heart, see whether you can use the power of your mind to slow your heartbeat down, just a touch. Just see whether you can use the power of your mind to slow that heartbeat down just a little.

You might find that in slowing your heartbeat down, your whole body has, in turn, slowed down as well, becoming lazier and lazier. Know that you've got absolutely nothing whatsoever to do now except relax. There's nobody wanting anything from you, nobody expecting anything from you, so you can allow your whole body to just continue to relax.

Feel how the rhythm of your heartbeat is smooth, steady, and effortless. Smoothly, easily, quietly, comfortably, it is beating. Now become aware of the rest of your body—your hands, arms, and so on. Become gradually more aware of your whole self—aware of your hands and arms, sensing how they are now, aware of your legs and feet as well. Again just sense how relaxed they might be, and wonder if it's possible to relax them even more. Get so in touch with yourself that you can actually get your whole body, perhaps, to relax even more, yet remain totally alert. Notice now how even your face muscles can begin to relax. Relax and let go of those tensions that were there, almost, but not quite, completely unnoticed. Become aware of the skin and the muscles of your face settling, smoothing out. It is a good feeling. Wonder just how long all that tension was there, where it all came from in the first place, and then realize that you simply couldn't care less as you feel it draining away from you now. See how good it feels as you continue to sense the beating of your heart and the absolute steadiness of your body's rhythm. Remain so absolutely relaxed and comfortable that you simply can't be bothered to even try to move even one single muscle even though you know you easily could if you wanted to. I know that you easily could if you wanted to, but you simply can't be bothered to even try. Allow yourself to just be relaxed and relax even more now. Be as lazy and relaxed as anyone could ever wish to be. Say to yourself, I wonder if I can now manage to relax even more even though I am already as relaxed as it is possible for most people to ever be.

Find the last tiny traces of tension in your body and simply let them go with each easy, gentle breath you breathe. Allow every muscle, every fiber, every cell of your entire body to be as beautifully relaxed as anyone could ever wish to be.

Hypnotherapy

A suggestible person in an alpha or a theta state can be guided by a therapist, with the client's permission, to transcend or shift out of certain negative, depressive, obsessive-compulsive patterns; reduce certain fear and phobias; reduce pain reactions and stress; and even change what, at one time, were considered involuntary physical responses. There are many misconceptions about hypnosis that are promoted in popular culture. One is that somehow the hypnotist can make you do something that is against your will. Note here that hypnosis is nothing to be feared. A hypnotherapist cannot make you do or believe something that you do not wish to.

Among the most skilled practitioners of alpha and theta induction are medical hypnotherapists and certified clinical hypnotherapists. Hypnotherapy is distinct from what is commonly known as stage hypnosis—the type of hypnosis performed as entertainment in nightclubs. Therapeutic hypnosis has always been a valuable tool in the hands of a skilled practitioner.

Hypnotherapy can generate relaxation through deep breathing, slow the heartbeat, and create a sense of emotional balance—all important results in the treatment of depression when it is associated with panic and anxiety. Once a person is in a voluntarily suggestive state, hypnotic suggestions can replace catastrophic thoughts with a more grounded, healthier thought process. Hypnosis may even help a person remember the origins of the depression and begin to understand the causative event from a new perspective.

Hypnosis is best used as part of an integrated therapeutic approach to the treatment of depression. It should never be used to replace counseling, nutritional therapy, or medication. If anything, hypnosis can help the process of healing move along more smoothly and quickly. Working with a professional hypnotherapist will help you develop a sense of personal vision, define achievable goals, and choose a path to take you in the right direction. It will help you to transcend despair, rediscover hope, and become fully alive.

Counseling and Psychotherapy

Beginning with Freud, many therapies have focused on a patient's family or personal history. The main benefit they offer is that they may help the patient understand the source of their depression. However, knowing the cause of a problem does not necessarily offer a solution to the problem. Exploring the past through therapy and counseling-based workshops or seminars may be very helpful, and should be considered as part of any program in order to heal depression.

Leo Buscaglia, the popular motivational author and lecturer, defined six ages in a person's development. These stages are infancy, childhood, adolescence, maturity, intimacy, and old age. There is a level of wisdom and effective behavioral patterns that exist in each of these age domains. When a person has not developed the appropriate patterns for each stage, depression may arise. In such a situation, counseling and psychotherapy may be of great value.

One of the earliest approaches for the treatment of depression was through psychotherapy. Psychotherapy consists of a client speaking with a professional (sometimes but not always licensed), who supports and guides the client or patient to gain insights about him- or herself. These insights encourage the client to make positive changes in feelings, behavior, and daily living habits. As popular as antidepressant medication has become in the last half of the twentieth century in treating depression, controlled research studies have shown that, in many cases, psychotherapy was as effective as medication in reducing—and even eliminating—symptoms of depression.

There are many forms of psychotherapy and counseling. In almost all approaches, the goal of the counselor or therapist would be to help the client or patient understand the underlying cause of the depression and, of course, overcome it. Studies indicate that counseling can be as effective as antidepressant medication in treating chronic, moderate anxiety states, as well as simple phobias and depression.

There are a wide range of psychotherapists and counselors to seek out for help. They include psychiatrists, psychologists, social workers, and specially trained therapists such as family therapists, pastoral counselors, behavioral therapists, Gestalt therapists, and body-mind therapists (those that integrate hands-on healing with counseling). All therapy and counseling techniques and systems involve suggestibility as part of the process. Psychotherapy and mental health counseling comes in many forms ranging from Freudian and Jungian psychoanalysis, Gestalt psychology, rational emotive therapy; Ericksonian hypnosis (and its offshoot, neurolinguistic programming), inner-child work, and family therapy. Whatever approach you choose, it is important that you enter some type of counseling as part of your overall healing program.

A skilled therapist should have a background in the study of human development and personality; interpersonal, marriage, family, and group-community dynamics; cultural systems; research methods, and supervised field experience.

Cognitive-Behavioral Therapy

Dysthymia is a mild but long-lasting form of depression. People with dysthymia are usually able to carry on with their daily activities, including their jobs, but the depression can linger for two years or more. There are a number of psychotherapeutic techniques that have been found to be helpful in the treatment of dysthymia. Most of these approaches are relatively brief and focus on reversing the self-defeating behavior and negative thinking that are common in this type of depression. The two most popular—and the ones receiving the most attention from researchers—are interpersonal therapy, developed by the late Dr. Gerald L. Klerman at Cornell, and cognitive-behavioral therapy (CBT), developed by Dr. Aaron Beck at the University of Pennsylvania in Philadelphia.

Cognitive function includes a wide range of processes, none of which are considered conscious action: perceiving, judging, calculating, and thinking are all unconscious actions. The goal in CBT is to modify your behavior. The techniques used in CBT are based, in part, on exploring the influence our perception has on our sense of who we are and how the questions we ask ourselves shape our perception. This approach is often successful, and much of the current research being conducted on counseling techniques for depression is focusing on CBT.

The focus of treatment in CBT is directed at defining and organizing the patient's basic beliefs, and showing how those beliefs support and recreate the patient's dysfunctional patterns. For example, "Since I am a victim, the things that happen to me are not my fault." An approach to CBT, known as systemic desensitization, focuses on showing patients techniques for relaxing major muscle groups as the patient is brought progressively into closer contact with a feared object, say an insect.

Treatment usually consists of weekly sessions and lasts a few months. During this period, discussions take place between the patient and the therapist, and the patient is given both behavioral and written homework to complete.

CBT has some similarities with other psychotherapeutic approaches including psychodynamic therapy. A key difference is that CBT sessions

are more structured and the cognitive therapist is more active and direc-
tive. The content of the sessions is focused on exploring and testing cognitive distortions and basic beliefs of the patient.

Because learning theory forms the basis for behavior therapy, depressed individuals who have deficits in social skills owing to poor social
role models, or who have a history of learning difficulties, may especially
be helped by this approach. Integrating training in social skills, modification of self-destructive thinking and behavior patterns, scheduled activities, and modifying attitudinal patterns and irrational thoughts are used
until the depression dissipates.

It should be mentioned that factors such as the process of aging, environmental toxins, and vitamin and mineral deficiencies can negatively
influence all of these actions. In fact, research indicates that various nutrients, including antioxidants such as CoQ10 and flavonoids (polyphe-
nolic compounds with antioxidant effects), can improve cognitive function,
probably because antioxidants combat the free radicals that have been
implicated as the cause of brain damage. This theory was tested on elderly patients by a group of Canadian scientists who gave them vitamin
supplements and trace elements. The result was improved cognitive function in the supplement group in comparison to the placebo group.[4]

Interpersonal Therapy

In interpersonal therapy, treatment usually consists of weekly sessions lasting about four to six months. The goal here is for the patient to
recognize connections between mood changes and what is happening in
his or her life. The therapist may help the patient explore specific areas
of difficulty such as role transitions including divorce and job loss, grief,
conflicts in the workplace or home, and the inability of an individual to
initiate or sustain social, professional, platonic, or romantic relationships.

Pastoral Counseling

Pastoral counselors are trained in both psychology and theology; thus
they can address various aspects of psychologically and spiritually based
depression. Pastoral counselors are found in every major Protestant denomination, as well as the Roman Catholic and Jewish faiths, and other
belief systems such as Unity. They will work with people of faiths different from their own. However, in practice, clients often prefer to work

with a pastoral counselor who shares their faith, membership in a specific denomination within a faith, and general beliefs. There are also many types of counseling and psychotherapy based on the worldview or philosophy specific to a religious tradition. For example, there is a type of psychotherapy based on the Buddhist philosophy.

In initial meetings, the subject of faith should be raised to assure that client and pastoral counselor are comfortable with each other's perspective. A pastoral counselor may be able to help you address these matters in the context of religion and spirituality. Since they are not physicians or nutritionists, they will generally not be skilled or qualified to monitor your medication nor can they design an herbal or nutritional program.

Have no fear that a pastoral counselor will try to convert you to a specific faith or belief. Pastoral counseling is very much the same as any other type of counseling you might seek from a psychotherapist except that counselors also have training in issues of spirituality and faith. The mission of an effective pastoral counselor is to allow clients to grow into the fullest people they can be, not to convert anyone or preach to anyone about their beliefs. Whatever your beliefs may be, a pastoral counselor will help you integrate what you believe into how you resolve your current problems.

Pastoral counseling works with persons from all different faith traditions, and persons who espouse no faith tradition. Whether you are Buddhist, Methodist, Jewish, Muslim, Hindu, Jainist, Christian, or athiest, you are welcome at most pastoral counseling centers, and your beliefs will be respected. In some cases, pastoral counselors have more education than other mental health professionals. For example, some pastoral counselors at the Fellow level in the American Association of Pastoral Counselors have completed a three-year Master of Divinity program, plus an additional degree or equivalent of four years of graduate academic work. In comparison, licensed clinical social workers have completed a two-year Master of Social Work degree beyond undergraduate coursework.

To find a pastoral counselor, check if your community is served by an accredited or affiliated pastoral-counseling center. These centers offer a number of certified pastoral counselors working in different religious traditions with whom you can meet. If you are unable to locate such a counselor in your community, you can call the American Association of Pastoral Counselors at 703-385-6967 to find the name of a certified pastoral counselor near you.

Most pastoral counseling centers are not-for-profit, and pastoral counselors often work for modest fees, which are generally lower than those charged by other traditionally trained mental health care professionals. It is the prevailing ethic of pastoral counseling that every effort is made to treat everyone, regardless of ability to pay.

Spiritual Counseling

Like art, love, and philosophical truth, spirituality cannot be easily defined. Sometimes we become overwhelmed in our attempt to understand our place in the world or in the larger workings of the universe. The attempt to understand nature or know God is a response to this experience that can appear as confusion, depression, or wonder. Though commitment to organized religious practice has diminished over the last few decades, the interest in spirituality has actually increased.[5]

For some individuals, spirituality is the experience of being moved to wonder. It describes certain enlivening feelings that come unexpectedly into our consciousness. Spirituality is concerned with the affairs of the divine nature and is inherently irrational. Nevertheless it is no less valid than a scientific view of things and is an essential element of the human experience.

There are a number of approaches that can be taken to address depression tied to emotional spiritual issues. For example, you can read sacred texts such as the Bible, the Koran, the Buddhist Sutras, the Bagavad Gita, the Guru Granth Sahib, and other spiritually oriented literature, especially writings that help add spirituality to everyday life. Three of my favorites are *Care of the Soul* by Thomas Moore (Perennial, 1994), *The Road Less Traveled* by M. Scott Peck (Touchstone Books, 2003), and *Zen Flesh, Zen Bones*, compiled by Paul Reps and Nyogen Senzaki (Shambhala, 1994).

You can join a spiritually based support group or discussion group that addresses religious or spiritual issues or join a house of worship in your community. You can also listen to spiritually based motivational tapes.

You can seek out a life coach, mentor, or spiritual counselor. These counselors are not licensed and not necessarily certified, but there are very talented individuals who serve in this capacity. To locate a coach or mentor, seek the support of people you trust and care about.

As discussed in the previous section, you can seek out a pastoral counselor. Pastoral counselors are trained mental health professionals and, as such, work with individuals, families, and groups. The nature of the therapy is agreed upon by the client and pastoral counselor.

Finally, you can pray daily or whenever you are moved to do so.

Somatic Psychology

Developed by Stanley Keleman, somatic psychology is a simple yet profound approach based on the belief that panic and depression are so connected, they are actually "two sides of the same coin." Both depression and panic, as well as the different gradations in the emotional continuum extending between them, are marked by characteristic physical patterns adopted by the body. Generally speaking, the panicked body is rigid, as if "paralyzed with fear," and the depressed body is flaccid and collapsing, as if drowning in helplessness and apathy. These physical patterns arise unconsciously in response to emotional events.

Keleman's pioneering work includes a series of movements and exercises that are intended to magnify or dramatize the characteristic physical patterns, then to systematically undo them in order to influence the correlated emotions. The goal of the movements is not to make you feel better, but to magnify your capacity to self-manage your physical-emotional experience and to return your sense of self-potency. The exercises can be performed lying down, sitting up, or standing. Each one is done twice, the first time with the focus on the way the body is held and the second time with the focus on the emotions.

To learn more about somatic psychology, see the videotape *The Shapes of Depression and Panic: Simple Exercises to Help Manage Depression and Panic*, produced by Stanley Keleman and led by Terrance McClure. This fifty-nine-minute tape costs $24.95 and is available from Center Press, 2045 Francisco Street, Berkeley, CA 94709.

Eye Movement Desensitization and Reprocessing

Eye movement desensitization and reprocessing (EMDR) is a technique that reduces fears by requiring clients to imagine traumatic events in a gradual fashion in the presence of a supportive therapist. It is used in the treatment of a wide variety of mental and emotional problems, including various phobias, post-traumatic stress disorder, and learning disorders.

The method, developed by Francine Shapiro, Ph.D., involves visual imagery, which is a key element of many behavioral therapies. In EMDR, the client is asked to recall a traumatic event in great detail, then to think of the predominant image or emotion connected with that event while simultaneously following the therapist's finger as it is passed back and forth in front of his or her eyes. The goal is to reduce the stress associated with the memory of the traumatic event.

Neurotherapy

Neurotherapy, also known as neurofeedback, is a behavior modification approach using EEG biofeedback equipment to increase voluntary control over the amplitude and pattern of various brain wave frequencies. It is based on the theory that the brain has four main frequencies: delta, theta, alpha, and beta. Using the EEG equipment, the client is taught to identify when a particular brain wave pattern is occurring and how to regulate it.

Caution

No matter which form of therapy you choose, don't become dependent on your therapist. There is good support and bad support. Therapists are not gods. They are there to help you. Some are better than others, as in all professions. If you go to a psychiatrist or psychologist, especially one that diagnoses psychiatric disease, remember that these diagnoses are interpretations of your own illness experience and that these interpretations are themselves cultural products. The goal of effective therapy is to enable you to be in touch with your emotions in a healthy, productive way and to enable you to interact with the world effectively.

Music and Sound

Humans have always been fascinated by the way music (which is, in part, a succession of rhythmic auditory signals) and other rhythmic sounds influence the mind. Specific instruments, rhythmic noises, and repetitive sounds are used in many religious and spiritual traditions as mind-altering and brain-training tools.

When the human body comes into contact with sound, a resonance occurs and the body's cells are affected. Depending on its origin, resonance is the process whereby a primary vibration initiates a secondary vibration, which then becomes harmonious with it as each begins resonating at the same frequency. Resonance can be experienced in a destructive form when an operatic voice holding a note with enough intensity and length shatters a wineglass.

Sound is the constant motion of energy as it vibrates and resonates. Every sound is composed of three important interconnecting elements: pulse, wave, and form. None of these can exist without the other, and together they create a singular powerful force. This energy field has electromagnetic qualities that travel through the body's "wireless anatomy pathways," feeding and sustaining every cell in the body, and all of the organs, glands, muscles, and nerves composed of these cells. If in some way this energy supply is interrupted, then the key processes for sustaining life are interrupted as well.

In the early 1960s, Andrew Neher, a researcher investigating the effects of drumming on EEG patterns, found that rhythmic pounding dramatically altered brain wave activity. Other researchers have found that drums at frequencies in the theta wave EEG frequency range (3 to 7 cycles per second) were predominant during shamanic initiation rituals.

When a composer creates a piece of music, he or she is manipulating the frequency of the rhythms and tone of the music. This is often done with the conscious and intentional goal of influencing the brain states of listeners.

Cultures from ancient to modern have used music and sound to ease melancholy, alter moods, and lift the spirit. We all intuitively know the power of music and sound. When we are down or depressed, we can play music that is uplifting. When we are sluggish, we can play music that gets us up and going. And we all know how important music is in creating the right mood for romance.

In 1980 Dr. Thomas Budzynski, a clinician and biofeedback researcher conducting a preliminary study of an early sound and light machine, found, "Results rendered from production of drowsy, hypnagogic-like states (with theta frequency used), to vivid, holograph-like images. At times, images from childhood were experienced." Budzynski called the machine a "Facilitator of Unconscious Retrieval" and a "Hypnotic Facilitator," and he wrote of the therapeutic benefits such a device might have since it seemed "to allow the subject to recall past childhood events with a high degree of being there quality."[6]

Budzynski points out that if sound and light could actively induce a state of deactivation in which the brain is passive, but not asleep; awake, but not involved with the clutter of an ongoing existence; then "it may be a state in which new cognitive strategies could be designed and developed." He also points out:

> If we can help a person to experience different brain-wave states consciously through driving them with external stimulation, we may facilitate the individual's ability to allow more variations in their functioning through the breakup of patterns at the neural level. This may help them develop the ability to shift gears or "shuttle" and move them away from habit patterns of behavior to become more flexible and creative, and to develop more elegant strategies of functioning.[7]

In recent years sound-light devices have been developed that can create and combine a seemingly unlimited array of beat patterns, chords, and tones; as well as allow the choosing of many different light-flash intensities and patterns. Some devices can be preprogrammed at just the push of a button or the flipping of a switch to stimulate certain states of consciousness, including certain types of meditation, sleep, and extreme alertness.

Mind tools have been highly effective at producing states of profound relaxation and awareness. In the 1930s, scientists began to study the effects of rhythmic light and sound on the brain. They discovered that the brain's electrical rhythms tend to assume the same pattern as a flashing light stimulus. Research since that time has shown that deep states of relaxation can be quickly produced with light-sound devices, and these devices may also increase suggestibility and receptivity to new information. The importance of this in the treatment of certain types of depression is enormous. A therapist skilled at the use of light-sound machines can quickly stimulate the desired brain wave state.

In the late 1940s, W. Gray Walter, a highly respected British neuroscientist, used advanced EEG equipment and an electric strobe light to explore what he called the "flicker phenomenon." Walter wrote:

> The rhythmic series of flashes appear to be breaking down some of the physiologic barriers between different regions of the brain. This means the stimulus of flicker received by the visual projection area of the cortex was breaking bounds, its ripples were overflowing into other areas.[8]

In essence, Walter had discovered that rhythmic flashing lights quickly altered brain wave activity, producing deep relaxation, precise and clear mental images, and a trance-like state. He also discovered that the flickering seemed to alter the brain wave activity of the whole cortex instead of just the areas associated with vision.

Vibration and Nitric Oxide

In 1998, Robert F. Furchgott, Louis J. Ingnarro, and Ferid Murad made a discovery that changed medicine. They discovered that our cells produce and release a gas called nitric oxide. Their discovery was so important that they won the Nobel Prize in Medicine and so significant that the U.S. government and the pharmaceutical medical complex has spent over $200 million investigating nitric oxide. Nitric oxide has been determined to aid in the development of the auditory system and participate in cochlear blood and is additionally responsible for the induced exhibited physiological effects.

The immune system uses nitric oxide in fighting tumors as well as viral, bacterial, and parasitic infections. Nitric oxide transmits messages between nerve cells, is a mediator in inflammation and rheumatism, and is associated with the processes of feeling pain, sleeping, learning, memory, and possibly depression.

Today landmark research is shedding new light on how music and sound affect depression and our moods. In 2002, George Stefano, Ph.D., and John Beaulieu, Ph.D., made a revolutionary discovery: Vibration transferred to cells by using tuning forks causes the cells to spike nitric oxide, setting off a cascading of physiological events that directly influence our state of mind. By understanding nitric oxide, we can establish a scientific link between biochemistry, medicine, and music and sound healing. A tuning fork is a sound instrument that is calibrated to an exact cycle per second. A tuning fork consists of a stem and two prongs. When they are sounded, the prongs vibrate back and forth, creating a precise tone.

This was an important discovery for those involved in alternative medicine as well, for one of the ways many practitioners of energy-vibrational medicine unblock energy is through the therapeutic use of tuning forks. With tuning fork therapy a healthy, balancing process of resonance occurs.

By gently tapping the tuning fork and applying the sound generated by the tuning forks on various areas of the body, a new beneficial pattern forms and unbalanced detrimental patterns are eliminated. The sound generated by the tuning fork affects both the conscious and the unconscious mind, especially on an emotional level.

The discovery of this nitric oxide factor served as a type of bridge between mainstream scientific research and the application of that research in the field of healing and wellness. Nitric oxide is a molecule created by a nitrogen atom bound to an oxygen atom. It is made in our cells and released into the surrounding tissues as a gas.

Scientists use many vibrational terms to describe the behavior of nitric oxide. The release of nitric oxide by our cells is termed *puffing* and is used to describe the rising and falling of the nitric oxide gas. The rising or outgoing phase of puffing sends a signal to our cells to relax. The falling or inward phase of puffing tells our cells to wake up and be active.

Flatlining is a term used to describe the absence of nitric oxide puffing in our cells. Flatlined nitric oxide is the body's cellular response to psychological and physiological stress. In an ideal world we would quickly adapt to stress and our nitric oxide would continue puffing. If the stress continues and our nitric oxide levels continue to flatline, we will experience increasing levels of depression. Recently Cell Dynamics, a private laboratory conducting research on nitric oxide and its role in sound, herbology, and meditation, published research showing that different tissues puff nitric oxide in different rhythms.

When our nitric oxide is spiked, we immediately feel better, endorphins are released, and we get a powerful sense of well-being. Simultaneously nitric oxide acts to balance our autonomic nervous system, allowing us to come into a state of balance. This positively affects serotonin levels in our brain, which then lifts our mood.

Tuning forks spike nitric oxide. Research demonstrates that when tuning forks are placed on bone or connective tissue, they resonate throughout our whole body, causing flatlined cells to spike nitric oxide. Research further suggests that listening to tuning forks as well as special music will spike nitric oxide. The implications of this research in both the medical and the energy paradigms are profound.

Our body is like a resonance chamber. Researchers reporting in the *Journal of Acoustical Society of America* found that connective tissues conduct vibration. They proved that the degree of resonance in distant connective tissue sites was directly related to the frequency of the sound that stimulated it. In other words, the vibration of a tuning fork placed on top of the head can be measured at the big toe. Our whole body vibrates with the tone.

This research suggests that being in the right rhythm, saying the right words, and listening to good music can vibrate our whole body, spike nitric oxide, and lift depression. Research also has proven that tuning forks can tune people like musical instruments. When we are tuned to the correct tone, our cells vibrate in resonance with the sound and our bodies create just the right chemicals for our mental health. Duke Ellington had the right idea when he sang, "It don't mean a thing if you ain't got that swing."

Research is now yielding over 3,000 papers on nitric oxide a year. The remarkable role nitric oxide plays as a messenger between nerve cells was revealed by John Garthwaite and colleagues at Liverpool University, who first identified it in the brain. Subsequent measurements have shown that the brain contained more of the nitric oxide synthase enzyme than any other organ.

The use of music as a means of inducing positive emotions and subsequent relaxation has been studied extensively by researchers. A great deal of this research has centered on the use of music as a means of reducing feelings of anxiety and stress as well as aiding in the relief of numerous pathologies. The precise mechanism responsible for these mediated effects has never been truly determined. Many researchers believe that nitric oxide is the molecule chiefly responsible for these physiological and psychological relaxing effects. Furthermore, this molecule's importance extends beyond the mechanistic, and is required for the development of the very process that it mediates.

Tuning Forks

Those who work with tuning forks may do so using different approaches. Some practitioners work with fourteen forks, each tuned to the vibrational frequencies associated with each of the key meridians (energy pathways in the body) of the Chinese medical system. Other systems express a direct relationship of a musical note to a specific gland, chakra (healing center in the body), or color.

The sound produced by the vibration of a tuning fork is called the fundamental note. In addition to this note, there are other notes called harmonics or overtones, which are sounded simultaneously. The more tuning forks are sounded, the more vibrational frequencies there are. In addition to the two frequencies one experiences from two different tuning forks, there is a third frequency that is actually the difference in tone between the two tuning forks. This third frequency is known as an interval. So with just two tuning forks, the body is actually responding to three vibrational frequencies.

When multiple forks are sounded, the effect is a multitude of different frequencies, overtones, and harmonics administered to the body as a cornucopia of sound. Specific tuning fork techniques are used on the cranial bones, the jaw, the spinal vertebrae, and the nervous system and muscle reflex areas. Many practitioners use a specialized tuning fork known as an Otto Tuning Fork. An Otto Tuning Fork is a normal tuning fork with weights added to the prongs. The weights cause the tuning fork to transmit more vibration through the stem. For this reason, these tuning forks are excellent for placing directly on the body.

Otto Tuning Forks are available in three frequencies: 32, 64, and 128 hertz, or cycles per second. Tuning forks are precise instruments and therefore we need to know exactly how many times they vibrate in one second. For example, if your tuning fork says 128 hertz, then this means that the prongs move back and forth 128 times in one second. The higher the hertz, or cycles per second, the higher the pitch of the sound, and conversely the lower the number, the lower the pitch of the sound. From among the three Otto Tuning Forks, I recommend using the Otto Tuner 128.

To sound your Otto Tuner 128, hold it by the stem and tap the flat side of the weights on your knees or the palm of your hand. To determine how much pressure to use, press the tuning fork onto one of your knuckles. Make contact with the base of the stem and gently press until you feel the vibration being transferred to your body. Experiment with different pressures. Start lightly and then gradually increase until you feel the maximum vibration.

The following is a good protocol to use with the Otto Tuner 128 to help relieve depression. Perform the protocol sitting down and in a place where you feel safe. Before you tap the tuning fork, take three deep breaths and relax. If you wish, visualize light or something positive as you breathe. When performing the protocol, all areas are general because the vibration travels through the entire cranium.

1. Press the Otto Tuner 128 to the back of your head, in the area of a little bump called the occipital cranial protuberence. Press no more than three times.
2. Press the Otto Tuner 128 to the center of the top of your head. Press no more than three times.

3. Press the Otto Tuner 128 behind your left ear, in the area called the mastoid process.
4. Press the Otto Tuner 128 behind your right ear, in the mastoid process.
5. Press the Otto Tuner 128 to the center of your forehead just above your eyebrows, to the area known as the third eye in yoga.
6. Press the Otto Tuner 128 to your chest or sternum one time.
7. Take a deep breath, and relax for one minute or more.

Caution: If you have a history of osteoporosis or have a fracture, do not press the Otto Tuner 128 to your bones. If you have a pacemaker, do not press the Otto Tuner 128 to your sternum. In general, if you feel any pain when pressing the Otto Tuner 128 to bone or soft tissue, then do not continue to press.

Another good tuning fork to use is actually a set made by Body Tuner. The set consists of two tuning forks, a C 256 hertz fork and a G 384 hertz fork, which make the interval of a fifth. The interval is called a fifth because in our Western musical scale, C and G are exactly five notes apart.

Lao Tzu referred to the fifth as the sound of universal harmony between the forces of yin and yang. In India, the fifth is believed to create a sound through which Shiva calls Shakti to the dance of life. Apollo, the Greek god of music and healing, plucked the fifth on his sacred lyre to call dolphin messengers to Delphi, where they channeled messages to the oracles.

The alchemists called the interval of a fifth *crux ansata*, and considered it to be a transition point where matter crossed over into spirit. In the crux ansata, also called the *ankh* by the Egyptians, there is a still point where the earth ends and our ascension into spirit begins. For them, the number 5 was numerologically the perfect combination of even 2 and odd 3, representing the unity of heaven and earth.

The fifth is a general sound tonic. Some of the benefits of the fifth are that it lifts depression, increases joint mobility, balances earth with spirit, and acts as a general tonic. It directly stimulates nitric oxide release and has antibacterial, antiviral, and immune-enhancing properties; balances the heart and pituitary gland; and releases opiate and cannoboid receptor sites in the third brain ventricle. It also balances the sphenoid bone and the sympathetic and parasympathic nervous systems.

To use the Body Tuner tuning forks, hold the tuning forks by the stems with moderate pressure; not too tight and not too loose. Do not hold your tuning forks by the prongs because the prongs need to vibrate in order to create the sound. Gently tap the flat side of the tuning forks on your kneecap. Do not hit your kneecap. All it takes is a gentle firm tap and your tuning fork will sound. It is best to tap your C 256 fork first on one knee and then your G 384 fork on your other knee. Bring the forks slowly to your ears, about three to six inches from your ear canal, and listen to the sounds. *Note*: If you do not want to tap the forks on your knees, then you can tap them on a carpet.

Find a safe quiet place and tap your tuning forks and slowly bring them to your ears. Let yourself go into the sound like a meditation. When the sound stops, lower your tuning forks and wait at least fifteen seconds before sounding them again. You can sound them up to seven times.

Another method of using your tuning forks is to learn to hum their sound. Tap them on your knees and bring them to your ears. While listening to the sound, take a deep breath and softly hum until the sound of your humming resonates with the sound of the tuning forks.

Your goal is to create a humming anchor sound that you can hum at any time without having to have your tuning forks available. When you hum the sounds of C and G without having to sound the tuning forks, it is called toning.

Breathing

Until the last few decades of the twentieth century, the mechanics of breathing and the relationship of breathing to respiratory muscles had been largely ignored or misunderstood. Massage and healing touch are often associated with reducing depression because touch has a healing and balancing quality for the emotions as well as the body. The meeting place of touch, the heart, body, mind, and soul is through energetic-vibrational centers known in Ayurvedic medicine and numerous other Eastern healing systems as the chakras. There are many different approaches that one can use to free up those areas where repressed emotions are stored. The use of guided breathing and intense sound is among the most effective. Stress in immoderate quantities overloads the body's resources and can be very harmful. If the body cannot handle the stress overload, it may reach a "pathological" tension. When this tension increases, your breathing may become very shallow. Shallow breathing has a pronounced effect on the blood circulation throughout the body and reduces the amount of oxygen that reaches the brain. In addition to shallow breathing, your muscles will tighten up, especially around your pelvis, neck, and shoulders. This chain of events can lead to depression.

Though breathing is an automatic action, the quality of how a person breathes is not. Emotions, physical patterns, and response to the environment all influence the manner in which a person breathes. Sadly, most individuals have unbalanced, emotionally restricted breathing patterns.

When you breathe deeply and exhale forcefully or scream repeatedly, a deep emotional release may take place. This release takes place in convulsive waves that begin in the pelvis and spread out throughout the body in orgasm-like waves. When guided breathing is done as part of an "emotional release bodywork" session, the client may be asked to act out his or her physical or emotional pain with the face, voice, or body. In time, this may trigger memories and release early emotional traumas.

As you are breathing deeply and using sound as a release factor, it may be very helpful to make unusual faces. Often a set facial expression will be a part of the individual's body armor (the storage of past emotional traumas in the muscle tissue and fascia as cellular memory). For example, someone who smiles when relating tragic events may be blocking his or her true feelings. If you are working with a partner, you can have him or her push on your chest while making different sounds or screaming.

Artistic Expression

Certain approaches to healing, especially meditation, visualization, art, and prayer, are internalized forms of expression. They are part of an inner journey involving emotion, visions, imagery, and feelings. This path can be called a journey of the spirit or soul or a connection with divine energy. However we name this process, it deeply involves a type of healing that comes to us from within our own resources.

Scientific research has shown that art—both creating it and viewing or experiencing it—can affect every cell in the body, instantly creating a physiological shift that changes the immune system, alters blood flow to all the organs, and increases healing. Many forms of art, including dance, music, painting, and sculpture, heal by not only changing a person's emotions, attitudes, perceptions, and emotional responses to the world but also by changing their physiology. Art can shift a person's neurotransmitter levels and brain wave patterns, and affect their autonomic nervous system. Art affects every body cell, instantly creating physiological changes especially in the immune system and circulation to all the organs.

Neurophysiologists know that prayer and art are associated with similar mind-body changes and brain wave patterns, as well as being deeply connected in meaning and feeling.

Art can heal by changing a person's physiology and attitude and bring an individual from a state of stress, fear, sadness, and depression to one of deep relaxation, inspiration, motivation, and creativity. Scientific studies show that art and music can create hope and strength in dealing with emotional challenges, especially depression.

Prayer

There is a general trend throughout the country toward spiritual and religious practice though not always in the most formal of ways. For many people, prayer without specific ritual or ceremony is the closest way they connect to the "divine." This spiritual trend shows up in diverse ways, including the popularity of Marianne Williamson's writings and lectures, the *Chicken Soup for the Soul* book series, and the general movement toward a more holistic approach to healthcare. People are examining their lives more, and prayer is the spiritual side of this self-examination.

The most popular spokesperson on the power of prayer to the scientific community is Larry Dossey, M.D. He is the former chief of staff of Humana Medical City in Dallas and was cochairman of the Panel on Mind/Body Interventions at the Office of Alternative Medicine at the National Institute of Health.

Dr. Dossey stresses a number of factors concerning prayer. He believes that:

- Love is more of a factor in effective prayer than religious belief.
- The influence of prayer and meditation on the human body is indistinguishable.
- Negative prayer should be avoided. This would include curses, hexes, and angry thoughts. The key is to pray with love as a guiding motive.

When a person feels buried under the weight of depression and seems lost in an ever more complex world filled with multiple priorities and confusion, it is often difficult to know what one needs to have. Many people are perceived to be highly successful and yet they are depressed as they struggle at a job that is not satisfying to them and in relationships that do not meet their basic emotional needs. The one defining factor that they can use to create joy and abundance in their lives is an experience or a connection with what we might call "the divine power." Through this connection, real or imagined, a person may come to experience a sense of love and respect. Love and respect can manifest in many forms but on a basic level they involve communicating our needs, doing things which are physically and emotionally healthy such as exercising regularly, eating well, meditating, getting enough sleep, and surrounding ourselves with people who are kind, loving, nurturing, and supportive. We must take care of our spiritual needs, whatever they may be—and prayer is a key way of addressing these needs. Prayer is important not because God requires it, but rather because we do. The act of praying is a sacrament. It is a conscious, experiential event of an inner divine presence or intent.

Prayer can be a call to the spirit world and to spirit guides and angels for help, verbal acknowledgment of one's relationship to the spirits, or a statement of appreciation for grace received.

Most people think of prayer as asking God for a favor. This is certainly one type of prayer. One can use prayer as a source of moral comfort, as a response to moral challenge, as an appreciation of gifts received, as an acknowledgment that we are challenged, or as an acknowledgment that we are never given more than we can handle. It can even be viewed as a means for connecting to your spirit guides and angels. One form of prayer is to surrender to the divine wisdom while asking for nothing in return. This surrender is considered in certain religious traditions to be the most sacred of relationships with the divine power. Some have found this "surrender through prayer" to be the ultimate healing tool. In the end, even seemingly unanswered prayers can be a vehicle for healing.

To pray is to be immersed in a sense of divine love. It is to tap into your inner truth, the truth that lies above the mental state. In true prayer you enter an altered state of consciousness. You forget your mind, your body, and your own ego; and connect to the divine consciousness.

Sometimes when we are in doubt, grief, or fear, we can create closure with a loving and nurturing prayer such as the following: "I thank the divine force for giving me the opportunity to serve my partner selflessly; if it be the Lord's will, may this session open doors of love and healing for him/her."

There is no one way to pray. It is not how you pray that counts but how the prayer affects you. Studies conducted by Herbert Benson of Harvard University Medical School, who also produced important research on meditation and relaxation, show that telling someone that there is "one right way" to pray can disenfranchise people from praying and produce "prayer drop-outs."[9]

Meditation and Visualization

"Look at that emptiness. There is brightness in an empty room. Good luck dwells in calmness. If there is not (inner) calm, your mind will be dancing about though you are sitting still. Allow your ears and eyes to communicate within but shut out all knowledge from the mind."

—Chuang Tsu[10]

An important aspect of exercise and depression is the increased amount of oxygen that exercise brings to the brain through the circulation. It is known that oxygen relaxes nerves and muscles, and carbon dioxide tenses nerves and muscles. As we have already discussed, in order to maximize the intake of oxygen, it is essential that you breathe fully and diaphragmatically. Remember to completely exhale as much of the air from your lungs as possible.

Meditation is both the simplest and the most complex of processes. In meditation, a person may be in a state of contemplation, musing, or reflection. He or she ponders, is lost in thought or is focused on a thought, empties the mind or fills the mind with imagery, evaluates, examines, and much more. This is all done in a quiet environment, usually in a sitting position.

Meditation is a form of mental sense impressions. Many mental health professionals have used inspirational skills, visual imagery exercises, and communication and meditation skills in combination to rapidly increase individual awareness and effectiveness. By using visual imagery, these practitioners have found that their students become more emotionally and physically receptive and that benefits are recognizable almost immediately. The beneficial response to meditation techniques has been especially pronounced for individuals under tremendous stress or who have a sense of helplessness, hopelessness, and isolation.

Meditation can increase self-confidence and feelings of connection to others. Many studies have shown that depressed people feel much better after a meditation session. Although meditation has been found to be very helpful in bringing relief from depression, some, more introspective forms of meditation are not always appropriate as a therapeutic tool. This is especially so in those clients who experience a constant sense of self-loathing. Some individuals have reported that attempting to focus inwardly can sometime intensify a sense of despair, negativity, hopelessness, and despondency. Though some specifically introspective meditation techniques may be of value for some depressed individuals, it is best not to use these for clinically depressed individuals, especially if they are in the midst of a depressed episode where they are harboring thoughts of self-harm.

There are, however, therapeutic meditation techniques that enable the depressed patient to consciously balance his or her nervous system and channel mental and emotional imbalance into calm, safe, restful, and harmonious directions. Meditation is not always a pleasant experience. As noted writer and teacher Joan Borysenko notes:

> Meditation may lead to a breakdown of screen memories so that early childhood abuse episodes and other traumas suddenly flood the mind, making the patient temporarily more anxious until these traumas are healed. Many so-called meditation exercises are actually forms of imagery and visualization that are extraordinarily useful in healing old traumas, confronting death anxieties, finishing "old business," learning to forgive, and enhancing self-esteem.[11]

The Value of Meditation in Treating Depression

Meditation reduces depression, in part, by training the mind to redirect its focus away from thoughts of depression and onto a fixed internal or external point. When doing an external meditation, a person can focus on a candle, a spot on the wall, or some other external point. Without cessation, meditators direct all of their mental faculties toward the point they have chosen.

When a person begins meditating, it is best to start with as little as five minutes in the morning and five minutes in the evening. As days go by, the time dedicated to this exercise should be increased to twenty minutes two or three times per day. Consistency and regularity of practice are the keys to success with meditation since, over time, it will condition the mind toward calmness and serenity.

This type of meditation is widespread throughout the world. It has even been studied at Harvard University. A good book to read if you want to know more about this type of meditation is *The Relaxation Response* by Herbert Benson, M.D. (Outlet, 1993).

Research at the University of Wales, and reported on ABC-TV *Online*, has shown that a combination of cognitive therapy and a Buddhist-influenced technique called "mindful meditation" can help prevent the recurrence of depression. Unlike more introspective types of meditation that can sometimes exaggerate a sense of despair and hopelessness, "mindful meditation" helps the depressed individual to be conscious of shifts in their thought patterns and maintain "balanced thinking patterns." Mindful meditation can become a valuable tool for a depressed individual in facing the fear, insecurity, disappointment, frustration, and anger that is often associated with this condition. According to an *Online* interview with Professor Mark Williams of the Department of Psychology, University of Wales, mindful meditation can reduce the chances of depression returning by 50 percent.

Professor Williams states:

> Mindfulness is a way of bringing you into the present moment and to invite you to sample what it's like when actually you come into the present moment and allow the thoughts and feelings and the tensions and the stresses and what your body's doing at the moment just to be what they are, and not to try and fix them or change them in any way.[12]

For a sample mindful meditation script, see "The Mindful Meditation of Eating a Grape" on page 168.

Another type of meditation that has been useful in reducing depression is what I call "intuitive creative meditation." This is the most common of the various types of meditation. It uses all of the memory senses—taste, smell, sight, and sound—as well as the intuitive faculties. In this technique, you actively visualize some scene or process with no end goal.

Here is a basic intuitive creative meditation: Imagine yourself walking along a path in the woods. You can sense the trees, hear the sound of the leaves. Walking along, you come to a waterfall. There is a path behind the waterfall that leads to a tunnel with a beautiful purple or violet light at the end of it. You walk into the tunnel. At the end of the tunnel is a bright healing light that bathes you and dissolves your depression.

Notice, in this meditation, that you are in touch with the details but there is no apparent end to the meditation. In this process, it is your job to create a positive environment where your inner voice can supply the missing pieces in your quest.

Some individuals do prefer meditating with a goal in mind. This is a technique used by everyone from high school athletes to successful business-minded people. In this technique, one imagines a goal that one wants to attain. This might be a world record or acceleration in healing and wellness. Then use the same approach as in intuitive creative meditation. However, at the end of this tunnel is an opening, and at the other end of the opening is the visual image of the goal achieved.

Remember: The intention of all our meditations is to create a healing bond between body, mind, and spirit, and to create an open space through which your inner voice may manifest.

The Mindful Meditation of Eating a Grape

In mindful meditation, you do not focus on your inner thoughts but rather on an action or an object. In an eating meditation, you might sit quietly and eat one grape while focusing your mind on that simple act.

1. Find a quiet place with a table and straight-backed chair where you will not be disturbed. Place a single grape on a plate on the table. Sit in the chair with both feet flat on the floor. Place your hands, palms up, resting on your knees.
2. Look at the grape for a minute or two.
3. Pick up the grape and place it in your mouth while focusing your attention on this action.
4. Slowly roll your tongue around the grape, feeling its shape and texture.
5. Slowly bite down on the grape, feeling the juice and experiencing the taste.
6. Slowly chew the grape. Focus on this action and the different sensations in your mouth.
7. Slowly swallow the grape. Focus on this action and the different sensations in the muscles of your throat.

8. Finish this meditation by taking a long deep breath. Exhale slowly and gradually. Remain quiet for a few minutes, becoming aware of your surroundings without getting up or moving around.
9. Slowly begin to wiggle your toes and fingers.
10. When you feel acclimated to the surrounding environment, you can arise.

How to Begin Meditating to End Depression

If you would like to begin meditating but don't know how, the best thing to do is to explore the different styles of meditation and see which, if any, seem appropriate for you. Start with five to twenty minutes twice daily, but if the depressive symptoms intensify, then stop. Consider working with an experienced meditation teacher. They can offer consistent, step-by-step guidance and feedback to help you feel more secure in your practice.

The evident power of meditation reinforces the concept that there is a direct relationship between the health of the body and the mind. When a person is in a balanced state of health, their life objectives and visions will be more clearly defined. With this clarity of thought and focus, the ability arises to act with greater effectiveness. This is so because, with this clarity, there is the knowledge that positive results are within reach.

Mental imagery and meditation play vital roles in all aspects of personal development both in the early creative and innovative phase and in later phases when innovation is applied through action. In articles and books about imagery and meditation, there is one fundamental point: As you think, so will you become.

Note: If you are a member of a particular religion and are concerned that meditation might be contrary to your faith, have no fear. There is nothing religious about meditation. It is simply an exercise in quieting the mind, balancing the nervous system, and supporting glandular function in returning to a correct state of hormonal balance. In the end, the benefit of meditation is the reduction and even elimination of depression.

Light and Color Therapy

The first demonstration that light is the source of color was conducted by Isaac Newton in 1666 when he produced the rainbow of hues of the visible spectrum by passing a beam of sunlight through a glass prism.

Phototherapy is the clinical use of light to treat various ailments. Color therapy is an art-science type of phototherapy based on the fact that physiologic functions respond to light and to specific colors. It is known that different colors give off different wavelength frequencies, which have different effects on physical and psychological functions. Many different health professionals have found the use of colors to be a valuable tool in the treatment of various physical and mental conditions, and in influencing health.

It is common sense to know that using colors in one's daily life influences how we feel. Certain choices of color will even promote a sense of inner harmony and peace of mind. With this in mind, researchers and psychologists have shown greater interest, through the years, in the ways that physiologic functions respond to specific colors. This has led to research on the effects of colored light on muscles. In one study, when subjects using a hand grip were exposed to red light, the electrical activity in them increased. When the test involved an increase in blue light, their grip lightened. Another report stated that when officials in England switched the color of bridges in London from black to blue, the rate of suicides jumping off the bridge was cut in half.

Research has shown that color-tinted eyeglasses can be highly effective in the treatment of learning difficulties, notably dyslexia, which has been found to be a causative factor in certain types of depression. This specific effect of color was first noted by psychologist Helen Irlen and confirmed by the British Medical Research Council.

When you see a color, you are not looking at a characteristic of a substance or an objective component. Color is a phenomenon of perception, a component of vision, and a psychophysical event consisting of the eyes' physical reaction to light, and the automatic interpretive response of the brain to wavelength characteristics of that light at a certain brightness level. (At lower levels, the eye is unable to make color distinctions.)

More than any physiological effect, color therapy predominantly affects the mind. Thus, it is important to use shades that bring joy, harmony, and serenity. The best colors for this purpose are white, gold, violet, and blue. Bright, loud, flashy, and artificial shades are sometimes useful when there is low or inert energy. Combinations of opposite colors can be too stimulating and irritating. Shades that are dull, dark, turbid, and muddy cause the mind and senses to become heavy, inert, and congested. Pink has had remarkable results in a number of environments. A color called "bubble gum pink" has calmed excitable mental patients and reduced the violent tendencies of prisoners.

It is only in the last few decades that structural studies have been done on the influence of light and color on brain function. Most of what is known about color is based on energetic-vibrational medicine, as well as ancient esoteric systems whose fundamental principles do not always merge well with the Western scientific tradition. Every scientist knows that every natural element of the Periodic Table—that's the table of elements you had to study in high school chemistry—has a specific color wave. For example, the characteristic color wave of oxygen is blue, whereas, hydrogen's is red. In certain circumstances, we see light passing through these different elements and experience them split into the prismatic colors.

Though it might seem that the influence of light and color is dependent on visual perception, this is not always so. Colors have different frequencies, some of which are not visible to the eyes. Light can be broken down into three primary colors: blue, green, and red. You can produce all of the colors of the spectrum, from white to black, by combining these three colors in different intensities. The human eyeball has three specific receptors that measure each of these three primary colors. The brain combines the information from these receptors into one multicolored image.

It is now accepted by most scientists that color need not be seen for it to have recognizable physical and psychological effects. The recognition of this phenomenon by researchers, referred to as eyeless sight, dermo-optic vision, or bio-introscopy, has come about from studies involving individuals who, though blind, colorblind, or blindfolded, were able to distinguish colors. Now we know that a blindfolded person will experience physiological reactions under different colored rays. It is as if the skin sees in Technicolor. Noted neuropsychologist Kurt Goldstein confirmed this. In his modern classic *The Organism*, he shows that not only can the skin be stimulated by contact with different colors, but such contact can also

produce different effects. He states that "it is probably not a false statement to say that a specific color stimulation is accompanied by a specific
response pattern of the entire organism."[13]

Research shows that certain areas of the skin are light sensitive and
also respond differently to different wavelengths (colors). Preliminary evidence points to the fact that different wavelengths may create a different response in the endocrine system, thus stimulating or reducing
hormone production and affecting the course of depression and other
emotional problems.

The early work on color and healing in the West was not done by scientists but rather by mystics and esoteric philosophers. One of the great
pioneers in the study of vibrational healing and color was the Austrian
philosopher and mystic Rudolph Steiner, who suggested that the vibrational qualities of certain colors might be amplified by certain forms,
shapes, and sounds. Other pioneers followed Steiner, including Theo Gim-
bel and Max Luscher.

Many color therapists have explored the role of clothing designs,
room designs, and sound as keys to understanding the link between harmonics and the wavelengths emanating from different colors. The growing popularity of feng shui (the Chinese art of environmental design and
form) has added a new, non-Western dimension to this inquiry.

Combinations of certain colors, sounds, and shapes might be healing
or destructive. Research has also been done on the effect of color on the
autonomic nervous system and the treatment of hypertension. Dr. Harry
Wohlfarth found that respiration, pulse, and blood pressure rates decrease progressively under the influence of green, then blue, and finally
black light. This was important news for those suffering from stress-
based depression.

In recent years, research has shown that certain colors possessing a
longer wavelength can penetrate tissues deeper than other colors. This
information has been key in the development of technology that uses
color sensitivity to both diagnose and treat certain diseases, including
cancer.

How Color Heals

Consciously choosing your color schemes in clothing can help reduce
depression. Yellow, white, and turquoise blue are happier colors than brown,
dark blue, red, black, and gray. However, yellow may actually aggravate

depression in some individuals. This may be because more light is reflected by bright colors, resulting in excessive stimulation of the eyes. Therefore, yellow may be an eye irritant.

How a color is administered will depend on whether or not it is visible or invisible to the eye. The basic theory accepted by most color therapists, both scientific and energetic in orientation, is that, in the same way that people need certain nutrients, they also need to have contact with certain energetic wavelengths. These specific wavelengths manifest as color.

The visual system can make out many thousands of hues through the use of just three color receptors: one tuned to red, another to blue, and the third to green. Being deficient in contact with any one color means that you will be deficient in the precise wavelengths that color represents. Such a deficiency will affect you on many levels, including brain wave patterns, hormonally and emotionally. What is the solution? The deficient individual should be given that color in a specific way, at a specific time, in order to gain the best results.

Current research is focusing on the ways certain types of light interact with the human body, affecting metabolic, endocrine, and hormonal processes.

Beginning from the hypothalamus, a long and complex series of events take place that ultimately influence the pineal gland. As recently as twenty-five years ago, the pineal gland (which controls the daily rhythms of life) was thought by many researchers to be dormant. It is now known to secrete the hormone melatonin. Melatonin (which the body converts from serotonin) influences the functioning of every cell in the body. Research has shown that shifts in the timing, intensity, and wavelength of light control the conversion of serotonin to melatonin in the pineal gland. A deficiency of light can cause many problems, including interfering with the induction of enzymes required for melatonin production. Melatonin helps the body synchronize its functioning with diurnal, lunar, and seasonal variations. It also modifies many essential bodily functions, including those of the pancreas and the adrenal, pituitary, thyroid, pineal, and thymus glands. When light rays enter through the eyes (or the skin), they travel through neurological pathways to these glands. Different colors give off different wavelength frequencies, which have different effects on the physical and psychological functions of these glands.

Color is the energy of a light frequency. Whether we are aware of it or not, this frequency directly affects our minds in many ways, some obvi-

ously and others more subtly. Common sense tells us that there is a biological interaction of humans with light and color and that color can influence attitude and behavior. Various pastel colors have been used for
years to paint walls in schools and prisons because they seem to control
moods and behaviors in a more positive direction than other colors. Stage
lighting is used in the theater because it is common knowledge that different colors can influence the emotional and physical response of the
audience.

One of the great pioneers in understanding the influence of color on
humans was the New Jersey–based medical doctor–attorney Dinshah
Jhahdiali, who called his work in this area "Spectre-Chrome Therapy." I
had the opportunity to know his son, Jay, himself a pioneer and writer on
veganism and vegetarianism. Jay told me of how his father had published
extensively on the subject of color and healing, and had been violently
persecuted and prosecuted for his ideas. Sadly, the ignorance and resistance of some ordinary minds is not limited to nutrition and the persecu-
tion of holistic doctors but has extended to many other areas of healing as
well.

It is essential that we understand that we are not only biochemical or-
ganisms but also spiritual, emotional, and structural beings. It is not just
food that affects our biochemistry but also water, air, sound, smell, touch,
and light.

How to Use Color Therapy

According to information presented on the Internet by Nicole Pascal
Motivational Designs, "The influence of colors on a person can be greatly
enhanced if delivered by means of designs that combine colors with specific shapes."[14]

Color therapy can be applied through a variety of ways including through
colored light and color pigments (such as paints or swatches). Incorporate
color therapy by choosing specific colors for your clothing, towels, and
colored lights; using blocks of color; coloring or drawing with crayons;
and using specific color pigments in paints and swatches. Color is also
effective in visual imagery. Here is some information to consider:

- Consciously choose the colors of your surrounding environment.
  This can include your car (interior and exterior), home furnish-
  ings, clothing, work space, bedroom, and living room.

- Use color consciously in lighting all key living and working areas. You can use colored lightbulbs or place colored glass over light-bulbs.
- Close your eyes and visualize colors or meditate on colored man-dalas (brightly colored patterns used in India and Tibet as part of meditation practice).
- Create an art project using stained glass.
- Use full-spectrum lights in the winter to alleviate SAD. If you do not have access to full-spectrum lights, use soft lights instead of fluorescent or neon.
- Generally speaking, choose mild and harmonious shades.
- Choose colors that you might associate with nature and harmony: flowers such as red roses, white lilies, and yellow daisies and sun-flowers; green trees, grasses, leaves, and shrubs; the turquoise blue ocean and the blue sky.

To bring color into your life, experience the color change of leaves in autumn. Notice the scarlet-red leaves on the maple trees and the bright yellow oak leaves. If you can, plant fresh, multicolored flowers in your garden. Gardening is itself therapeutic. Keep fresh-cut, colorful flowers in your home.

It could be said that when a person is deeply depressed, the color has gone out of his or her life. The goal of all emotional healing—and specif-ically color therapy—is to return the rainbow into the depressed individ-ual's life and keep it there.

Colors and Their Attributes

Certain colors remind us of past memories—some pleasant, others not so pleasant. Used effectively, color can excite, energize, inspire, mo-tivate, and awaken lost sensuality and sexuality. Each person must explore colors and their hues and see how he or she responds to each aspect of any color.

Working with color can be a subtle process. One cannot just say, for instance, that green does this or that because there are many types of green. There is jade green, lime green, olive green, and so on. Most greens are helpful for those suffering from anxiety, neurological imbal-ances, and depression. Green relaxes and soothes. Green with a yellow tinge tends to be very healing for those of a deeply intellectual bent who suffer from depression. These same people should avoid orange-yellow if they are individuals who think compulsively about problems down to the deepest detail while ignoring important aspects of healthy functioning.

Basic red, orange, and especially yellow can be used to stimulate a depressed person who feels paralyzed emotionally and can barely get out of bed. Red light appears to help athletes who need short, quick bursts of energy. Red is a great color for stimulating brain wave activity, and in stimulating the sexual glands. However, red also increases heart rate, respiration, and blood pressure, and should not be used therapeutically for someone with bipolar disorder.

Orange is a warm color and is great for expanding creativity, vitality, and sexual expression. It, like red, energizes and stimulates appetite and the digestive system. Orange and bright yellow, like red, may be too stimulating for someone suffering from bipolar disorder.

Yellow has an energizing effect on the nervous system. It improves memory and stimulates the appetite of those who have lost it while in depression. Since yellow helps improve memory, it is a good color to work with if you are engaging in journal writing as part of your healing process. It is for this reason that journal writing is best done on a yellow legal pad.

Yellow light has been shown, in some studies, to help reduce the symptoms of hypoglycemia. However, yellow should be kept in the background of color choices for those in the throes of a manic episode.

Pink is a good choice for balancing manic behavior. It appears that, when in pink surroundings, people cannot be aggressive, even if they want to, because the color saps unbalanced energy. Pink has been found to have a tranquilizing and calming effect within minutes of exposure. It suppresses hostile, aggressive, and anxious behavior.

Blue is also a good choice for balancing a manic pattern. Blue light can assist in creating a response requiring a steadier emotional pattern and energy output. This color has a calming effect, decreasing respiration and lowering blood pressure. Studies have shown that when disruptive children were placed in blue classrooms, their aggressive behavior diminished dramatically.

Translucent blue is not only calming but supportive of those who have a difficult time communicating their feelings. Blue stimulates inspiration and trust in your intuition. It lessens extreme suffering, especially in times of transition from a depressed to an active state.

In certain cultures, some colors are seen as being of greater benefit to a particular gender. Though red, orange, yellow, blue, and green are useful for both men and women, silver, in many cultures, is seen as a specific reflection of feminine energy. After childbirth, silver is used to balance the "mother" (yin) energy and feminine aspects of the personality.

Gold is considered to reflect the masculine energy expansive aspect (known as yang in energetic healing) of creation. The cosmic "father" energy can be used to balance the male factor in you.

Purple is the color most associated with prayer and spiritual inquiry, and can offer a key role in the process of healing depression. Violet has a similar association with spirit for many people, and may provide a sense of balance for depressed individuals who overeat in response to their depression. It also assists in reducing migraine headaches.

There may be times when it is not clear about which color is best, especially if a person goes through constant mood swings. In such a case, green is the best choice. A blend of warm and cool green is the best all-purpose healer to choose. It is soothing, relaxing (mentally as well as physically), and helpful to those suffering from depression, anxiety, or nervousness.

All color is an expression of energy vibrating. We live in a universe made of vibration and energy. The ability to distinguish and sense different energies is a fundamental property of life forms, and every living creature has developed ways to sense various types of energy and to either benefit from them or protect themselves from them. Within our bodies and emotions, energy storms occur constantly. This flowing energy comes into our consciousness through what we call the chakras. The chakras do not exist physically. They are subtle "life fields" that vibrate at specific frequencies and dynamically shift in subtle sounds, shapes, and colors. Generally speaking, they serve as the connections between the life force in our physical, emotional, and spiritual bodies and the unnamable divine energy that fills the entire universe. In the following chapter, we will explore in greater depth the role of energy in the healing of depression.

9 ✦ Vibrational Healing

Quantum physics has shown that everything in the universe consists of vibrational fields. Energetic-vibrational approaches to healing integrate many different approaches toward healing the body, mind, spirit, and even the external environment. Chinese medicine, for example, may use herbs, acupressure, acupuncture, and even feng shui to bring balance to various energetic pathways known as meridians. In fact, acupuncture has actually produced some positive results in reducing depression, usually taking about ten treatments to produce substantial benefits.

In this chapter, we will discuss the vibrational healing concepts of the chakras, chi, prana, and cellular memory, as well as the diagnostic technique of applied kinesiology and the treatment techniques of hands-on healing and vagus nerve stimulation.

Cellular Memory

Many physicists believe that all living cells emit biophotons. These energetic fields regulate every anatomical and physiological function. Dr. Deepak Chopra, in his book *Quantum Healing* (Bantam, 1990), described the concept that suppressed negative emotions such as stress and trauma are often stored as "cellular or phantom memories" in cells throughout our body. These cellular memories influence us energetically or vibrationally throughout years—even decades—which eventually cause emotional and physical illness.

When emotions that have been buried and supposedly long forgotten once again come to the surface, they can cause unexpected internal conflict, rage, resentment, regret, expectation, fear, disappointment, or depression. Some individuals are so traumatized at some point of their life that they have no means for expressing the emotional effects of this trauma. For such an individual to function emotionally, he or she must repress this trauma deeply into the vibrational pattern of the cells. This energy is transformed and transported to various organs and muscles, and is stored in them. Each muscle or organ expresses this repressed chi, or what Ayurvedic practitioners call *prana* energy, as physical or emotional imbalance.

The unaware individual may experience illness in the areas where the repressed energy is stored. For some individuals, the energy can remain repressed for years—dormant in organs, glands, or muscles—until some event or biochemical shift releases it. Though the cells of most organs regenerate, the cellular memories stored in them are constantly transferred to the new cells before the previous cells die. This cellular memory can block the flow of chi or prana. This blocked energy reduces the ability of new cells to release the memory of the previous dying or diseased cell.

Practitioners of energy medicine can determine, by reading the body, where these cellular memory blocks are. Techniques for doing this will vary from culture to culture and may include navel, face, and tongue analysis, as well as pulse reading and applied kinesiology-based techniques. Once an energetic-vibrational evaluation has been completed, there are many approaches to balancing and healing this released cellular memory.

There are a number of healing systems that claim to release deep cellular memories, thus helping the depressed individual to release long-held emotional and physical blocks. Among the most popular approaches are mind-expanding methods such as meditation and visualization; energetic healing processes such as polarity therapy and chakra balancing; and emotional and physical release or healing through hands-on bodywork techniques such as Reiki, the more aggressive hands-on Rolfing treatment, or the nonintrusive Feldenkrais Method, which works on the concept that if the body does not feel threatened—which is achieved with gentle, nurturing touch and moving of the body by the practitioner—the body will relax and feel safe so it can release pent-up emotions and memories.

The concept of cellular memory is difficult for many psychiatrists and psychologists to understand. This is unfortunate, since research in the field of psychoneuroimmunology supports the theory that our thought patterns instantaneously and directly influence immunity and other aspects of body chemistry. Even cellular biologists know that emotional trauma influences blood chemistry, and certain chemicals released into the bloodstream can block certain cell receptors in the body.

We live in a universe made of vibration and energy. The ability to distinguish and sense different energies is a fundamental property of life forms. Every living creature has developed ways to sense various types of both beneficial and damaging vibrational energy in order to survive. Human beings, however, have become more externalized in our focus. Our intellectual faculties have dominated our intuition. Thus, our vibrational sensitivities have been dulled.

Within our bodies, emotional energy storms occur constantly. This flowing energy comes into our consciousness through what we call *chakras*. The theory of chakras in America comes from the study of Ayurveda, in which equal importance is given to the body, the mind, and the spirit.

This is a concept that is somewhat at odds with Western approaches to the treatment of depression and other illnesses. The chakras do not exist physically. They are subtle "life fields" vibrating at specific frequencies and dynamically shifting in subtle sounds, shapes, and colors.

There are many popular descriptions of the chakras in New Age literature. Generally speaking, the chakras, or "energy wheels," serve as the connection between the life force in our physical, emotional, and spiritual bodies (chi, prana) and the unnamable divine energy that fills the entire universe (Tao in China, Shabd or Nam in India). In this sense, the chakras might be seen as possessing a spiritual quality. The concise descriptions that can be found in ancient yogic and tantric texts—many written in Sanskrit—speak of specific vibrational qualities that possess airy, fiery, watery, and earthy characteristics. A deep depression might be seen as an excessively earthy imbalance, whereas a manic state would be an imbalance of the air and fire chakras.

Chi Imbalance and Illness

Within all energetic-vibrational healing, there is a process of balancing antagonistic-complementary forces. When the circulation of chi (also known in Chinese medicine as ki or qi) is blocked or even lost, there is a disturbance of its flow to and from the organs. The result of this chi imbalance or depletion is physical and emotional imbalance. If the condition is extreme enough, various symptoms of illness may appear.

We may regain a balance of chi by absorbing external factors such as food, herbal medicine, aromatic oils, oxygen, light, sound, thoughts, and vibrations, and transforming these into prana or chi energy. In China, do-in therapy, acupuncture, tai chi, and qi gong exercises may be used therapeutically to either increase the production of, circulate, regulate, or calm the chi energy

As you develop your inner healing chi, you will begin to recognize that all healing comes out of a balance between the two cycles of motion and rest. This may even be seen as a balanced "energetic perspective" on bipolar disorder. Rather than the extremes of mania and depression, the alternating between expansion and contraction of chi in a balanced rhythmic sequence can cleanse internal and energetic toxins from the chi pathways and from the internal organs.

Diagnosing Chi Imbalance

The practitioners of traditional Chinese medicine and Ayurveda have turned the diagnosis of chi imbalance into a fine art. By examining the tongue and the eyes, tapping and listening to different parts of the body, and asking targeted questions, they can determine the type and degree of imbalance an individual is experiencing. In our modern Western culture, practitioners generally rely on four newer methods: applied kinesiology, thought field therapy, neuro emotional technique, and Nambudripad's allergy elimination technique.

Applied Kinesiology

Applied kinesiology (AK) is an energetic-vibrational system of analyzing the interactions between consciousness, organs, muscles, and acupuncture meridians. Developed by George Goodheart, D.C., in the 1960s, this approach is the foundation upon which many other healing systems are based.

AK in a sense connects Western and Eastern approaches to diagnosis and healing by teaching that every organ has an energetic relationship with a specific muscle. Thus an organ dysfunction is always associated with a specific muscle weakness.

Thus by AK muscle testing, the practitioner attempts to properly test the strength of a muscle in specific ways as a means of gaining information. This information may include the source of glandular imbalances, allergies, organ weakness, and many nutritional and biochemical imbalances. An AK practitioner may also place different substances in the patient's hand and test whether the arm can resist being pulled by the practitioner. If the arm is weak, this indicates that the substance causes an allergy or other physical or emotional problem. According to AK theory, an organ imbalance, an energetic imbalance in the meridian, a negative thought pattern, or a certain color or sound can influence the body and mind and thus influence the strength or weakness of a muscle.

An offshoot of AK that has become popular in recent years is a technique whereby the client imagines a thought or holds a food or other item, and rather than testing the muscle, the practitioner tests specific finger strength.

Critics of AK claim that scientific studies have never been conducted on this approach and that muscle test results may be too easily influenced by variations in the test technique, suggestibility, and muscle fatigue (from repeated testing). They also question how the number of pills held in the hand can somehow be registered and measured. Many AK practitioners claim to be able to specifically determine through a muscle test deficiencies even at very small levels. The idea that someone could do this without sophisticated tools, laboratory tests, or blood and urine analysis makes no sense to skeptics. I won't argue the point but will note that AK and offshoots of the system are extremely popular among highly respected segments of the alternative medicine and natural healing community.

Thought Field Therapy

Thought Field Therapy (TFT) is a system that integrates various techniques including AK-based muscle testing, voice analysis, and the "finger tapping" of specific acupressure points for the purpose of releasing blockages ("perturbations") of "body energy" associated with physical or emotional illness.

During a TFT session the practitioner may tap on these specific acupressure points—primarily located on the hands, face, and upper body—while the patient does repetitive activities such as repeating statements, rolling the eyes, or humming a tune. This may all be done as the client visualizes a distressing situation from the past. Developed by psychologist Roger J. Callahan, Ph.D., this approach "provides a code to nature's healing system." According to Dr. Callahan, it addresses the fundamental causes of these energy blockages, "balancing the body's energy system and allowing you to eliminate most negative emotions within minutes and promote the body's own healing ability."[1]

Neuro Emotional Technique

Neuro emotional technique (NET) is an energetic-vibrational system that combines aspects of visualization techniques and AK. The technique focuses on releasing a patient's emotional blocks, stored in the body's memory, through the use of AK, supplements, various energy-balancing techniques including homeopathy, and various meridian-balancing systems such as acupressure and acupuncture. It was developed by Scott Walker, a California-based chiropractor, who describes the technique as "a body-mind way, a non talk-it-out way, of dealing with emotional aberrations."[2] NET practitioners use AK muscle testing to "isolate a troublesome event." With the patient visualizing an image that he or she relates to the emotional state, the chiropractor adjusts the patient's spine or applies the other energy-balancing therapies.

Nambudripad's Allergy Elimination Technique

Nambudripad's Allergy Elimination Technique (NAET) is an energetically based system of diagnosis and treatment that uses muscle testing and other AK-based diagnostic approaches and acupressure and acupuncture to cure allergies. The theory at the base of NAET is that allergens cause blockages in the body's meridians. This energy blockage results in interference in the connection that the nervous system creates between the body and the brain. This blockage begins a chain reaction that ultimately results in an allergic reaction. By muscle testing various substances that have been placed in the hand of the patient, the NAET practitioner can isolate the source of the allergy.

Some NAET practitioners use an electrodiagnostic device that measures skin resistance to a small current emitted by the device. The treatment approach used in NAET involves the patient holding a sample of the allergen in his or her palm and touching it with the pads of the fingers while the practitioner applies acupressure on traditional acupuncture points using firm pressure applied by the hands or with a pressure device. Patients older than the age of ten may also receive acupressure or acupuncture on specific points on the front of the body.

Patients are then muscle-tested fifteen to twenty minutes later with the allergen again in their hand. If the process has been successful, the patient's arm should remain strong against the practitioner's pressure.

Patients are asked to avoid all contact with the allergen they have been treated for and are given a list of appropriate foods they can eat for the next twenty-five hours.

NAET may be of help to those who are experiencing depression related to allergies.

Hands-On Healing, Touch, and Massage

The experience of nurturing and healing touch is essential for mental health. Leo Buscaglia became famous for his hug therapy, and studies have found that people who do not receive touch and human contact have more infections and have imbalances in brain chemistry that can lead to depression.

Specialized forms of touch are important tools for ending depression. First, the cerebral cortex and thalamus identify a texture. This is then passed on to the limbic system, where it is decided whether you like how it feels or not. If it produces a sense of pleasure, it will affect the body and mind in other ways that can shift the biochemical imbalances that contribute to depression. In fact, the limbic lobe is where our emotions are stored. It is here where our memories are kept, and moods and desires are regulated.

This is why a simple odor can trigger a memory from childhood. For this reason alone, combining aromatherapy with hands-on healing can help heal depression.

Polarity therapy, Chinese acupressure, and various other hands-on healing techniques can sedate or stimulate energy centers in the emotions and the body.

According to Chinese medicine, depression may occur when the energy that feeds certain emotions, such as guilt or anger, is repressed. Pressing on depression-reducing reflex points can help to release this blocked energy. Once it is free to float to the surface, you can search these feelings and try to have a greater understanding of them.

For some important acupressure points that you can treat yourself to relieve depression, see "Acupressure Points for Depression" on pages 185–87.

Acupressure Points for Depression

The following are important acupressure points for relieving depression. You do not have to use all of the points. Using just one or two of them whenever you have a free hand can be effective in controlling your depression.

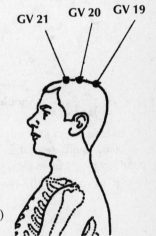

GV 21   GV 20   GV 19

Head Points:
The Posterior Summit (GV 19)
One Hundred Meeting Point (GV 20)
Anterior Summit (GV 21)

The head points are all located on the top of the head. Pressing them can relieve depression with accompanying headache and memory lapses.

Begin with the middle point, GV 20. Place your left thumb on the top of your left ear and your right thumb on the top of your right ear, then move the tips of your other fingers toward the top of your head and feel for a hollow near the top center of your head. This is where GV 20 is located.

GV 19, also situated in a hollow, and lies approximately one inch behind GV 20.

GV 21 lies one inch in front of GV 20.

As you apply steady, firm pressure to these points, relax your body and let your tension and depression slip away.

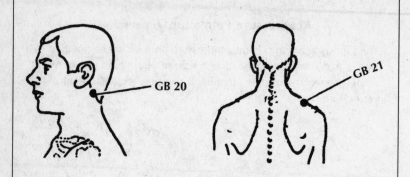

Wind Pond (GB 20)
Shoulder Well (GB 21)

GB 20 is found in the hollow between the two large neck muscles, just below the base of the skull. GB 21 is found on the top of the shoulder, two to three inches from the neck. Pressing them will help relieve depression with neck tension, headache, and irritability.

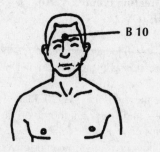

Heavenly Pillar (B 10)

B 10 is located about a half-inch from the base of the skull on the muscles bordering the spine. Pressing it can relieve the fatigue and emotional distress of depression.

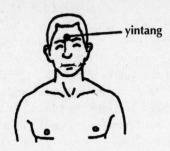

Third Eye Point (Yintang)

Yintang is located between the eyebrows in the groove where the bridge of your nose meets your forehead. Pressing this point soothes the emotions and relieves depression.

Vagus Nerve Energetic Stimulation

Research has also shown that functioning of the vagus nerve is an important aspect of emotional health, particularly in depression. When this nerve is stimulated, the functioning of the heart as well as the brain's emotion-sensing network improves.[3]

There are a number of hands-on techniquues that focus on the stimulation of this nerve energetically. Here is one that is done by a partner on the person with depression:

1. Have the person with depression lie on his or her back with legs flat and arms straight at the sides.
2. While you are standing at the end of the table or mat near the depressed person's head, gently cradle the head in the palms of your hands, with your fingers gently resting on the base of the skull. Do not massage the area or apply any pressure. The head should rest in your hands as if on a pillow. In a soft relaxing voice tell the person, "Relax your head completely in my hands."
3. Slide your hands on to the sides of the head with the ear on each side resting in between your thumb and index finger. This should

place your index finger automatically in a position that stimulates the reflexes to the vagus nerve. Direct the person with depression to place his or her hands on his or her abdomen and breathe deeply and rhythmically into this area three times, inhaling slowly to the count of nine and exhaling to the count of three. Hold this position for about three minutes.

4. Now guide the person with depression through this visualization: "Visualize the oxygen bringing relaxation into your body and exhale the tension out, feeling your muscles relaxing."

5. The person with depression may begin to feel warmth in your hands. When this happens, coordinate your breathing so the in-halation-exhalation patterns match. Close your eyes and repeat this breathing pattern for two to three minutes. Now remove your hands very slowly.

If the person with depression indicates in any way that he or she would like to hold this position for a while longer, return your hands. Do not remove your hands too quickly since this may be disquieting. This contact, when done properly, produces a sensation of having the entire body cradled and is extremely comforting.

All of the processes and techniques we have discussed in this chapter can lead to experiencing what is called a "state of flow." This is a positive experience for a person locked in the prison of depression. In a state of flow, you feel as if you have actually become one with the activity on which you are focusing. You may lose track of your body, emotions, sense of time, and even physical location. When you are giving everything you can to a particular vision or challenge, you become free of fear and anxiety. You have no room in your consciousness for boredom. Some people call it a "drug-free high," coming from the rhythm that seems to be part and parcel of working at the 100-percent level.

State of flow is not the type of concentration that creates great mental strain. When you are in a state of flow, you are in essence rowing along with a gentle, smooth-flowing stream, as opposed to trying to row up a waterfall. Through color, sound, hands-on healing, meditation, hypnosis, and the many other approaches to healing depression discussed in this chapter and this book, this "state of flow" becomes available to everyone. When a person can experience the state of flow, life becomes more joyous on every level and depression becomes a memory.

10 ❧ Maintaining Joy

"As our minds loosen their obsession with our practical affairs and everyday identities, we can open to glimpses of the inner peace that underlies our restlessness and discontent."

—Sarah Powers, "Answering the Call"[1]

Most of our daily activities are focused on experiencing immediate gratification. When we are thus gratified, we tend to be in a good mood. When gratification is unavailable, we may become impatient, cranky, and if frustrated enough, angry and then depressed. Because of this, much human endeavor is dedicated to controlling how we feel emotionally by means of various techniques, strategies, and chemical influences: exercise, food, coffee, meditation, dance, music, tobacco, alcohol, recreational drugs, meditation, hobbies, and so on. Some of these are healthy activities and others are not. They are all applied in our lives to give control of our feelings and moods from moment to moment.

Much in life is a conglomeration of random events and circumstances that lie outside of us, but our mood is a result of a combination of internal processes including glandular function, our unique biochemistry, our exercise habits, our sleep patterns, and more. It is also a result of our thinking. The depressed mind wants us to believe that its dark state is a logical reality when, in fact, it is a distortion of reality.

According to James Ray, an expert and speaker on success:

> Beliefs are nothing more than habitual thought. Thoughts, and the words we use to express them to ourselves, and others, have corresponding images in the mind. These images have corresponding emotions, the emotions have corresponding actions, and actions have corresponding results. So the path to any result is thought/word-emotion-action-result. If you want to improve the results you are getting, you must interrupt the habit of thought and create a new one.[2]

When you are consciously focused on harmony, love, friendship, spirituality, health, generosity, and detachment from the darker aspects of life, a new reality becomes apparent to the mind.

One of the great struggles of a mind trapped in depression is the constant attempt to define what is and what is not true. In the end, one can totally express and actualize what is true. The inherent difficulty of this struggle is that to know the truth, you must first know what is true. You must understand what makes something genuine, just, legitimate, or any of the other offerings in what might be a technical definition of truth. This is no easy matter.

Leo Tolstoy said, "Truth, like gold, is not to be obtained by its growth, but rather by washing away from it all that is not gold."[3] It is precisely through this process—the participation of the individual in the search for truth—that these insights are assured. The evidence is waiting for us but it does not appear immediately. In the process of realizing it, your depression will fall away like the cocoon of a caterpillar and you will emerge in flight as a butterfly.

The mind is a complex thing. It ascends quickly to what it believes to be the truth even if this perceived truth is based on hopelessness, fear, darkness, and despair. It is the nature of the mind to grab at any declaration, proposition, or alleged fact; it will create evidence to support its beliefs even if there is no personal knowledge to support this belief.

One process for coming out of deep depression requires the depressed individual to engage in an ongoing process of reducing attachment for negative thinking (what the Chinese call the "illusory self"). This is the self that intellectual knowledge tries to understand but is unable to. This often feeds into the type of attitude that contributes to depression. The good news is that as we learn to reduce the influence of this illusory self, so does the sense of despair so often associated with depression disappear. Through this process, the depressed individual realizes that attachment to the past and fear of the future are no longer relevant. In fact, this fear ceases to exist. At first, there is a distancing from all that was perceived as dark and negative. As the process continues, there is a detachment from ideas of despair and hopelessness and a focus on being present in living and experiencing all of the joy and beauty that is also available from life.

In this chapter, we will discuss the methods that people with depression have found to be helpful in reducing negative thinking, coming into the "now," and unearthing and experiencing the real and the joyful in life.

The Mind, Belief, and the Emotions

Throughout the healing process, there is a constant compensation between physical, emotional, and spiritual elements. It is this dance between energy and structure, spiritual and emotional, touch and movement, that makes the healing process so exciting, invigorating, and even fun. Whatever happens on one level of personal existence will reflect on all levels.

Every day scientists are surprised at the workings of the human mind. What seemed mysterious one day is obvious the next, and then some new piece of information arises to make it all mysterious again. At one point in time, a person may sincerely believe he or she knows something about something, and realize later that this information was completely inaccurate. Likewise another person may have great knowledge about something and not even be aware that he or she possesses such knowledge.

If an individual's depression is not the result of biochemical imbalances or genetics, then it may be the result of false beliefs or unproductive thinking. The generally accepted definition of a belief is the assent of the mind to the truth of a declaration, proposition, or alleged fact on the ground of evidence that is distinct from personal knowledge. Psychologists theorize (another term for believe) that many if not most of our beliefs come more from emotional need than rational deduction.

In fact, much of what we believe as a result of emotion becomes reality. Though we like to believe that we are for the most part logical beings, it is very difficult to get people to act in ways that are inconsistent with their innermost convictions and beliefs.

Your quality of life is probably based on your moods more than any other factor. No matter how wealthy you are, how good your job, or how physically attractive or talented you are, if your mood is not balanced and healthy, then every person, place, and thing that is part of your life will have a dark negative cloud over it. It is your mood that reflects both your physical and your psychological being. It is your mood that subtly defines the choices you make and the actions you take.

Affirmations

As you learn to use your intuition, it is essential that you remove what is often called *negative self-talking* from your internal conversation. Negative words such as *would, could, should, but, what if,* and *maybe* are not bad words; they just feed limited thinking and are of little value in helping the mind free itself from depression. Try to use inquiry words such as *who, what, why, where, when,* and *how.* In your private and public conversations, questions bring answers and answers bring freedom. You can also use proactive or neutral language such as: "I am unlimited possibility." "I can see the joy in living." "Contentment is my natural state."

Proactive statements of this type are called affirmations. Affirmations help create a sense of vision. Without a vision or a mission, life seems aimless. Think of something, anything, that excites you in a positive way. Art, sailing, philosophy, learning about history, making a difference in the world, your family. Now focus on ways that you can reach or fulfill that vision. A person with clear vision may be rich or poor but is deeply happy with his or her life while the person who has wealth or great material possessions but does not have a clear sense of vision or mission can be likened to a dog chasing its tail. Such people spend all their time worrying about getting more or keeping what they have, and they may become and remain depressed. There is absolute spiritual, physical, and emotional freedom for that person who has a clearly defined vision and an honest sense of who he or she is. The actual discrepancy between the vision and depression will create the fuel that moves an individual forward out of his or her depression, minute by minute, hour by hour, day by day, week by week, month by month, year by year. Without a vision or a mission, life seems aimless. Willpower and discipline without vision or a sense of purpose is struggle.

Following are nine affirmations that will help you to pass through situational depression. They are especially important for those who experience hopelessness and despair. Say these affirmations in the morning when you arise and at night before you go to sleep.

1. I deserve love and respect.
2. My ability to receive love is determined by what I believe I deserve to receive.
3. If I live with love in my heart, I always have enough of what I need.
4. I am never given more than I can handle. The support is always there either through grace or through the asking.
5. Everything in life involves change and transformation. Whether or not I choose transformation, everything is transformed by time.

6. My desire for habit and comfort is an essential part of the human condition. I will not judge myself for these desires.
7. At the moment I am ready, willing, and able to act on vision. It takes place spontaneously without discipline or willpower.
8. The fruition of my vision quest happens at the very moment that preparation and an opportunity meet.
9. I will never lose faith. I know there is always a light at the end of the tunnel.

Support Groups and Motivational Materials

One of the most important aspects to the healing of depression is never losing faith. You will eventually come out into the light at the end of the tunnel.

I recently spoke with one of my students, Rena Gordonson, about her own experience with depression and the role faith played in her own healing. Rena, a certified social worker in New York State, has had a particular interest in spiritual psychotherapy encompassing both Eastern and Western modalities and completed two years of postgraduate study in this area. Rena states:

> In February of 2000, a feeling of dread and hopelessness enveloped me that would change my life. I had become clinically depressed.
>
> My depression [the formal diagnosis was major depression and generalized anxiety disorder] did not manifest itself in a desire to stay in bed all day. I was usually up early and out of the house looking desperately for some relief in twelve-step meetings, the park, or with friends. But nothing could change the course of my illness.
>
> It got so bad that one night I just sat down on the pavement in the middle of the sidewalk and cried inconsolably. I also had suicidal thoughts that were neither mild nor fleeting. They were strong, powerful, realistic, and inviting.
>
> I eventually admitted myself into Mount Sinai Hospital, which led to Four Winds Hospital and a three-month stay at a treatment facility in Connecticut. When I left to go back home, I was nowhere near being healed.
>
> I did eventually heal with the help of doctors, medication, psychotherapy, friends, and family. I think the most important aspect of my healing was that I always had faith that my life could be better, and that if I was not able to hold that faith, the people around would do it for

me. I never gave up. Today, I still struggle with aspects of depression, but I think it is a normal level of depression. I do my best to eat properly, rest, and keep in contact with my therapist and friends, and I have just begun exercising regularly. It is said that addictions are a mental, physical, and spiritual disease, and I feel that the same can be said of depression.[4]

Positive, motivationally based thinking does make a difference! I often hear skeptics criticizing certain ideas as "fluff" and "pop psychology." My response to this? Different people heal in different ways, but clearly and without a doubt those with a view of life that creates room for hope, aliveness, and possibility are less depressed than those that see only despair, darkness, and hopelessness. Sometimes a simple story of a person overcoming seemingly insurmountable odds will help another person take that next step and make it through another day. Reading motivational books, listening to positive thinking tapes, and going to support groups can all help as part of a larger therapeutic program to heal depression.

Humor

According to the Association for Applied and Therapeutic Humor, *therapeutic humor* is "any intervention that promotes health and wellness by stimulating a playful discovery, expression or appreciation of the absurdity or incongruity of life's situations."

Many people were unaware of the power of humor to heal until they saw the movie *Patch Adams*—the true story of a medical doctor committed to using conscious joy and humor to heal. In the healing community, however, laughter has been known for years to have a curative effect on all types of physical and emotional illness including depression. Back in the 1970s Norman Cousins wrote *Anatomy of an Illness* (Bantam, 1991), a book that described his healing from an degenerative illness while sitting in a hotel room and watching comedy movies for hours on end and laughing until his sides hurt.

Laughter makes us less defensive about our insecurities, brings out our spontaneity, and is associated with the pleasurable emotions. Humor makes us feel lighthearted, joyous, childlike, and playful. It is virtually impossible to experience anxiety, fear, depression, or anger while laughing.

Laughter reduces stress hormones, increases tolerance to pain, stimulates breathing, and increases immune response by increasing healthy antibodies. Psychotherapists have begun integrating humor into the treatment of emotional and mental disorders.

A study at the University of Maryland Medical Center showed the healing power of a great "laugh." The study of 300 individuals, half of them heart patients, concluded that laughter could have specific, measurable physical and emotional benefits. "We know that anger and stress impair the endothelium—the protective barrier lining our blood vessels," says Michael Miller, M.D., who led the research team. "This can cause fat and cholesterol buildup in the coronary arteries. But laughter may have the opposite effect—it may stimulate elements that protect the endothelium."[5]

Humor has various cognitive effects. It can alter our perspective on life, reduce negative self-talk, change our mind-set from an objective, serious, logical sense of reality to a more creative, playful one. Laughter helps us to think in more flexible ways, "draw outside the lines," and function "outside of the box."

How do you use humor to get out of depression? Watch funny movies, read funny books, and watch the comedy station on television.

To learn more about Patch Adams and the Gesundheit Institute, as well as the Association for Applied and Therapeutic Humor, see "Resources" on page 224.

Mind Technology

Interest in how the mind works and advancements in technology have advanced at a rapid pace over the last fifty years so it was only natural for scientists to begin exploring ways that machines could be used to influence brain function and emotional states. Specialized machines including computerized light and sound units have been shown to produce quick and profound changes. Michael Hutchison's book *Mega Brain Power* (Hyperion, 1994) was one of the earliest and most important sources for exploring research in this field.

Since the original publication of *Mega Brain Power* in 1986, advances made possible through computer technology and new and more sophisticated combinations of sound and light are more valuable than ever in affecting brain function and depression.

Researcher Jill Ammon-Wexler, Ph.D., of the Innerspace Biofeedback and Therapy Center in Los Gatos, California, did a controlled study using a strobe light with color filters to provide rhythmic photic stimulation in variable frequencies and in selected wavelength or color bands. Working with twenty subjects suffering from phobias, she found that "remarkable resolution of the subject's phobic systems had occurred over the process of the 20 experimental sessions. There was also 'across the board' evidence for enhanced self-concept, and clinically-significant reductions in both anxiety and depression."[6]

Much of this research has brought us to a state where a simple machine and ever more advancing technology can be used to bring about a desired shifting of brain wave patterns and this can be achieved in minutes, even in people who have never had the experience before. Light and sound tools, in addition to meditation, hypnosis, and creative visualization, can help affect certain types of depression by reducing stress, increasing relaxation, changing negative attitudes and deep-seated behavior patterns, and even growing new connections in the brain.

Exercise

Exercise is key in treating depression. "Exercise creates chemical and psychological changes that improve your mental health." It may also change the levels of hormones in blood, elevate the beta-endorphins (mood-affecting brain chemicals), and improve the function of the autonomic nervous system.

Research indicates that exercise alters neurotransmitter levels in such a way as to reduce depression.[7] Exercise has also been shown to have cognitive effects. It reduces negative thoughts, alters people's perceptions of themselves in a positive way, provides an experience of personal mastery, and when practiced consistently, reduces symptoms of depression and prevents recurrences.[8]

Sadly, it is often difficult to motivate chronically depressed patients to expend the time and energy to regularly exercise. Walking briskly on a daily basis is a good way to begin.

Yoga stretching exercises are especially valuable for the depressed person because they involve practicing only as few as two or three poses taking just a few minutes. Coupled with balancing breath patterns, these postures not only provide a pleasant experience but also immediately help reduce the dark cloud of depression.

Dance and Movement Therapy

According to the Greek philosopher Plato, "Dancing is the one expression involving the faculties on all levels: spiritual, intellectual and physical." Dance has always been a highly expressive art form. Modern dance, which developed in the early part of the twentieth century, was particularly experimental and expressive, and less regimented than ballet. The natural progressive nature of this type of movement led to the realization that modern dance could be a highly effective tool when used to address issues related to communication and emotional expression.

Dance and movement therapy, which emerged from modern dance in the 1940s, has become a valuable tool for individuals of all ages who struggle to express their feelings verbally. To a trained observer, movement and dance reflect inner emotions. In fact, conscious changes in movement can also influence behavior. This is so in yoga and tai chi, and in dance and movement therapy. One of the greatest articulators of this concept was the late Israeli physicist Moshe Feldenkrais, who based an entire system of therapeutic movement on this observation.

Dance and movement therapists use a wide array of techniques to help the client cope with feelings of loss, encourage creativity, elevate self-esteem, and counter social withdrawal. The approach used will generally be based on the therapist's own background and the specific needs of the client. What most dance and movement therapists have in common is that they use a combination of unstructured and structured movements to support people to express their innermost feelings and conflicts without the use of words.

Dance and movement therapy can be conducted in individual sessions or in a group. Each is beneficial in its own way. Individual sessions are probably most desirable where the client would benefit most if the dance and movement therapist is able to observe the person portraying certain feelings or traumatic events through movement. Group sessions may be more effective when an individual has a history of social isolation. For such an individual, the sense of community and support and encouragement of other group members may help him or her open up more easily concerning emotional issues.

Some therapists "move with their patients in supportive and mirroring roles, while others act essentially as empathetic observers," says Dr. Fran J. Levy, a Brooklyn psychotherapist. "Occasionally, some therapists do their own dances to reflect what they perceive, or to help the group feel more comfortable with movement."9

Dance and movement therapy can help those suffering from a wide range of physical and emotional challenges, many of which are related to various types of depression. Some feelings are difficult or impossible to describe with words but can be expressed through movement. Family discord, personal psychological problems, and sexual issues can all lead to depression. By allowing a person to express and unfold his or her story through movement, the dance and movement therapist helps the client to release the emotional holding patterns that sustain depression.

Dance and movement are effective ways for a person to bring feelings to the surface, and identify and express them. In time, this expression may even take place through words. At this stage, talk therapy can be integrated into the process. As the process progresses, fear of communication and other barriers will fall away as the individual moves toward emotional healing and health.

Combined with meditation and visualization, dance and movement therapy can give a depressed person a clearer perspective of traumatic events or situations. A man might be depressed, for instance, because he feels responsible for some traumatic event that happened in the past. He may feel that somehow he could have prevented it from happening. By dancing or moving through an enactment of the traumatic event, the man can include various actions he imagines could have been taken. As the dance progresses, he might discover that there was nothing he could have done or that, if he had acted differently, an even worse outcome might have come about. The realizations and insights that come about through dance and movement therapy may enable the man to make peace with himself.

I had the opportunity to speak with dance teacher and Feldenkrais bodywork and movement practitioner Donna Gianell. She spoke about how the Feldenkrais Method helped her through a two-year depression. But before she knew of it, dance was Donna's means of healing when coping with death and a traumatic experience.

> Dance saved me as I watched my father die from cancer. Every day I watched him slip away. I was only fifteen. And my boyfriend broke up with me during that time, which didn't help. Nobody could really help. So I wore an emotional suit of armor for protection. Food was a major comforter. But when I danced, that heaviness was released and re-

placed with a dancer's "high." Through dance, I could express emotions of sadness, helplessness, frustration, and anger in positive, physical ways. And being able to control how my body moved through space psychologically translated into a feeling of control over my life.[10]

Dance was again Donna's therapy:

> . . . when I was hit by a car and suffered multiple injuries to my body and brain. After coming out of a coma, then having amnesia for a month in the hospital, my struggle to regain my life and sanity was indescribable. Doctors, psychotherapists, and physical therapists created a world of "You can't," "You're disabled," and "You will never be able to do—" I was hyperemotional, so conversations or situations were emotionally magnified, bigger than life.

Unfortunately, Donna did not have a healthy support system, and the situation worsened.

> Friends, family, and how I reacted to them fueled my depression. They were either undependable or had their own issues and viewpoints. Plus, I was constantly denigrating myself for things I had said when I was with them. I didn't sleep at night. I was thrown into a world I didn't understand with the maturity of a child, and I hated myself for it.
> After hating myself and being depressed for about a year, I wound up in the hospital with mononucleosis. Again, dance became my only hope. It was my rock, my security. It was my best friend and nonjudgmental. It was an oasis that I clung to dearly, turning away from physical and psychotherapy. I only danced. It grounded me and kept me from spiraling out of control.

When teaching dance to troubled children, teens, and adults with low self-esteem, accompanied with anger, frustration, and feelings of helplessness—even self-destructive actions—Donna says she witnessed their outlooks change to those of accomplishment, confidence, worthiness, joy, and hope.

> They focused on steps, movements, music—not on negative, debasing, and energy-depleting thoughts and emotions. And music sparked that desire to move, or maybe memories associated with the music, combined with the joyous and harmonious feeling of moving with the

music. So, through the discipline of dance, they—and I—found free-dom.

However, dance was not therapeutic for Donna when:

> . . . my mother, Ethel, and dance teacher and "designated mother," Georgia Copeland, died within six months of each other. I went into a two-year depression in the late nineties. Because dance had been such an integral part of my life with them, it now added to my depression. Fortunately, I had the Feldenkrais Awareness Through Movement [ATM] lessons, which helped by nurturing my body and mind. Moshe Feldenkrais said, "The way the body learns is through pleasure and ease." In ATM, you explore options of moving the body in effortless and enjoyable ways through verbal suggestions. Through this safe and nurturing physical method of communicating with the neuromuscular system, my negative emotions and views were replaced with ones of pleasure, fulfillment, choices, and hope. I could see options in life that I couldn't see before. That's why I took the training to be a Feldenkrais practitioner. It has done wonders for me, and I've seen it do wonders for those whom I have worked with.

"Feldenkrais ATM and dance free up the body and release tension through diversified movement, extending the body's range of motion, the blood circulation created from moving, and the joyous feelings experienced while moving," says Donna. "Organic bodies were not built for monotony nor were muscles created to be sat on or be sedentary. When that happens, our bodies hold and store emotions, which only add fuel to depression."

Rehearsals for Growth

Persons diagnosed with affective disorders typically present themselves as "being" depressed, anxious, or so on, thereby identifying themselves with their problems. Their worldview is shaped, both by themselves and by others, as reflecting a defect in their responses to life. A useful, alternative view is that such experienced affective states are social constructions, which can be altered through having novel experiences that are concurrently relabeled as nonpathological. Verbal-only therapies often lack sufficient impact to effect change in such clients, since their emphasis on relabeling experience fails to alter the familiar context in which the client concludes that he or she "is" depressed.

Developed in 1985, Rehearsals for Growth (RfG) is an application of theatrical improvisation to psychotherapy, most often with groups, couples, and families. RfG is not a stand-alone therapy but rather an approach that combines with most other psychotherapies. Clients in RfG are first offered improvisational exercises (unfamiliar tasks performed as themselves) and, later, improvisational games (both familiar and unfamiliar tasks performed as impersonated characters). Instead of using therapy to discover "who you are," RfG supports the exploration of "who else you could be," preparing clients to act heroically on the stage of life. As do other action (experiential) techniques, RfG opens alternative pathways of learning by deemphasizing verbal processing and heightening the use of emotional expressiveness and physical movement during sessions.

There are a number of features of RfG technique that make it effective in treating depression:

- The in-the-moment practice of improvising, which requires clients to think, emote, and move outside of their familiar habits and expectations.
- The shift in the social context of reality to a more playful and fantastic mode, thereby altering the usual affective climate associated with "being realistic."
- The construction of scenes that offer clients either the opportunity to explore novel solutions to a familiar social situation or the chance to contend with an unfamiliar one.
- The opportunity to play at being someone else, which gets clients unstuck more readily from habitual limitations, and thereby lessens the fear of, and responsibility for, exploring the consequences of change.

In an RfG Mood Change group of six to fifteen prescreened members, for example, sessions typically begin with a brief verbal go-around in which members report key choices in their real-life social performances that week. Next, everyone gets up from their chairs, stretching to warm up physically, then forming a circle and taking turns imitating each other's movements and expressions. At this point, the therapist offers one member the chance to enact a scene based on her or his earlier-reported key choice. If that member declines, other members volunteer to enact their key-choice scenes. All games and scenes are enacted onstage, an area set apart physically from where members sit as themselves. Group members are applauded generously for taking chances but are never shamed or pressured into taking the stage. Scenarios are loosely structured, sometimes by the entire group and at other times in consultation with the group members who play the main characters. Scripting of dialogue and action is minimal; players improvise most of the dialogue and are free to invent plot changes along the way, so long as these follow from what had previously been established within the scene. Following each enactment, players return to their real-life personae offstage and verbally process their work.

Most new members just watch initially, then volunteer to play minor roles in others' scenes. Group members are united by their efforts to discover and practice new ways of playing their roles. They encourage one another to take risks onstage, play supporting roles for one another, and share constructive feedback with one another about their effectiveness in the new roles.

Depressives often are first drawn to playing "extreme roles," such as extroverted or unrealistically cheerful caricatures. They try out playing these fearless and uninhibited characters, though once offstage, they revert quickly to emotional passivity. To deepen their onstage experience, the therapist occasionally interviews a client as a character he or she has played. The client's task during the interview is to hold to the character, improvising in-role. Group work is combined with "homework," which assigns elements of onstage behavior to be attempted in their everyday life to expand and integrate positive, expressive qualities into day-to-day social functioning.

As the work continues, client performances become more confident and nuanced. Those clients who make the greatest progress have internalized a vision of their lives as socially effective, enthusiastic persons bent on realizing that vision. Even those clients who have not been so active improve somewhat from participating in the group process.

Journal Writing

Journal writing is a therapeutic tool for problem solving, dealing with relationships, discovering and dialoguing the personal aspects of self, and developing positive affirmation messages as part of a strategy for improving self-esteem and self-worth. When you keep a journal, you have an opportunity to write about your feelings, especially the ones you are unable to express to others. They can be expressed as prose or through poetry. As in dance and movement therapy, you are able to express how you feel creatively. The more you express, the easier it is to climb out of the darkness of depression.

Social Skills

Individuals who suffer from depression often isolate themselves. This is a counterproductive pattern that only feeds the depression. Thus anything that reduces this isolation is recommended. First and foremost, when you see friends or acquaintances, start a conversation with them. If you do not generally run into people you know, try doing volunteer work. Volunteering is a great way to meet new people. To learn more about ways you can volunteer in your area, check out the Web at www.volunteermatch.org, go to your local Y, or talk to a local religious leader.

Another good way to meet new people is to join a house of worship. By attending services and getting involved in the social aspects of a church, temple, mosque, or other spiritual center, you will make new friends. Also consider taking a continuing education class or joining a club. To find something that interests you, check the bulletin boards in your local supermarket, health-food store, and wellness center. Contact your local college for a continuing education catalog.

If you are shy and hesitate speaking to people, try using Bach Flower Remedies to help reduce your shyness. Mimulus and larch are my favorites. See Chapter 7 for more information.

Stress-Management Plan

"Most people cannot emerge from really serious depression just by fighting; a really serious depression has to be treated, or it has to pass. But while you are being treated or waiting for it to pass, you have to keep up the fighting."
—Andrew Solomon[11]

The first step to freeing yourself of stress-based depression is to recognize that your goal is not eliminating stress but knowing when you've passed your stress threshold, then doing something about it. If you're overstressed, and you feel that your life responsibilities are making so much demand on you that you can't handle them much longer, then it's time to develop a personal, three-step stress-management plan.

First, find an off-the-job activity that gives you time off from stress. Relaxation and quiet time can work, as well as does physical activity in which you can release some of the tension you feel. Walking, jogging, tennis, and racquetball are all inexpensive activities that can give you a minivacation from the workplace. Once you find an activity that works well for you, make that a priority and commit yourself to one or two days a week at a specific time (or every day if you can manage it) that you will give to yourself.

Second, identify personal habits that intensify stress. This is harder to do. Try observing the ways in which you work. Are you a perfectionist, demanding too much of yourself and others? Do you rush through things that you might enjoy taking longer on—business or pleasure? Do you constantly worry about "what if" scenarios? Be aware of your feelings and note when you feel the most tense. Then think about what you are presently doing or what you were doing just previous to these stressful feelings. Is the stress self-imposed? How so? Once you've identified your stress-producing habits, write them down and keep the list handy so you can refer to it regularly. It will remind you to ease up and pace yourself.

Third, learn how to handle stressors. Look at your job and list the people, tasks, and environmental factors that cause you stress. Identify ten stressors that occur repeatedly and rank these in order of highest, most frequent stress to lowest. Then break down these general stressors into three categories: those you can eliminate, those you can decrease or modify, and those you cannot control. Now focus on the least powerful stressor in the first category; determine how to eliminate it, and do so. Then congratulate yourself. Don't you feel better already? Continue through that category, then move onto the second category and see what progress you can make on the stressors there. Keep a log of how you handled each stressor so that when others come along, you'll know how to deal with them.

The Sedona Method is a more structured stress-reduction program. It is a simple and highly effective technique for balancing the emotions and reducing the influence of physical and psychological stress. Seminars as well as taped programs are available. You may find them of great value, and this method is known to produce rapid and observable results. To order the Sedona Method program, see "Resources" on page 224.

* * *

As you can see, though there are many factors that determine a person's mental and emotional well-being, the one factor that is most within your control is the way you view life. If you have a poor attitude, everything will tend to seem negative and a source of fear. If you have an attitude that life is to be lived fully and in celebration, then even the sad and hard times will not get you down for any longer than it takes for some genuine introspection. In order to create abundance, it is important to have an attitude that breeds joy and success. I am not suggesting that you just start thinking positive. Though positive thinking is a wonderful concept, that is not what we are referring to here. You can certainly choose to see everything as positive but that will not help much while everything seems to be collapsing around you.

An attitude that creates productive and effective choices, without or in spite of fear and anxiety, involves the ability to see all things as possible even if you do not intellectually understand how this is so. There is great power in being able to see that possibilities are available even when you are not feeling positive. The key to this is a willingness to conceive of yourself as deserving all of the best that life has to offer. Having this outlook about things is not something that comes automatically at first. It is something that you develop over time and that can be taught to you. In time, how you think and see the world can have a major impact on your emotional state, especially your depression.

Depression is a thief, and the techniques, tools, and tips described in this chapter are a means of saving up and protecting your emotional valuables.

11 🏵 THE EMOTIONAL HEALING PROGRAM

Natural healing is a celebration of life and living. It is about the soaring of the human spirit; the inquiry into self; the surrender to wisdom, divine knowledge, love; the celebration and joy of being human; and the process of making a difference in the lives of others.

C. J. Jung theorized that a transformation of personality requires an understanding of, and making peace with, the unconscious. This includes its specific structures and active interactions as they become apparent during the process of achieving self-awareness.

The goal of the program described in this chapter is to reduce or eliminate the biochemical causes of depression or, when this is not possible, to at least prevent relapses. This is important, especially since statistics indicate that clinical depression tends to worsen with each subsequent attack.

An effective process to natural emotional healing can begin with an integration of herbs, nutrition, food supplements, meditation, prayer, and accupressure. Some of these approaches may be more attractive for you than others. The twelve-week plan that follows integrates many of these different approaches.

The theoretical basis for this approach is the commonsense view that a chain-link fence is only as strong as its weakest link—that is, that the most vulnerable point in any system (emotional, chemical, structural, mental, spiritual, familial) will be the first to reveal stress, and the way in which the stress appears is what we recognize as a symptom. This program is not for those who are suicidal or prone to physically hurting themselves. Such an individual should call the Suicide Prevention Hotline at 1-800-SUICIDE (800-784-2433). This hotline is manned by professionals experienced with this level of hopelessness and desperation.

Ultimately, the healing of depression requires a shift of the unconscious structures that shape and define ego-consciousness. With this shift, self-actualization begins to take place.

People all too often live their lives in regret of the past or with unrealistic expectations for the future, seeing each situation as an obstacle. Their thinking is dominated by thoughts of *what if, would, could, should,* and *maybe*. This is often what makes them ill and diseased. Natural healing is a vehicle for transforming this type of thinking. It is a process of possibilities. It is dedicated to inquiry into the who, what, where, why, when, which, and how aspects of human experience.

The twelve-week program presented in this chapter will show you how to integrate the best of the rational and the intuitive, to absorb the knowledge from the past and combine it with the best of modern technology, science, and current developments in human potential.

Week One: Review Your Lifestyle

In Week One, the goal is to explore the source of your depression. Do you have a deeply rooted biochemical imbalance that requires professional help? Have you been ignoring the fundamental requirements for emotional health? Review your sleeping patterns. Do you deprive yourself of sleep? Do you go to sleep with a busy mind, worrying about the past day? Do you get enough sunlight? Do you have a regular balanced exercise program? Do you use alcohol, recreational drugs, or tobacco products? Are you creative, and do you budget time for a creative project or artistic hobby such as dance, music, painting, or singing? Do you laugh and bring humor into your life? Do you engage in self-inquiry? The philosopher Aristotle stated, "The life unexamined is the life unlived." Do you have a spiritual component to your life? Do you begin and end each day with prayer, meditation, or the reading of sacred texts? Do you have a healthy emotional environment of supportive friends? Do you enjoy your job and the people you work with?

Depression if often the result of a life unfulfilled. If you live your life well and are still experiencing depression, or if you feel paralyzed to create a life of contentment, then seeking professional help may be the next step.

Week Two: Seek Professional Help

Once you have a sense that the source of your depression goes deeper than lifestyle factors, you should seek out a skilled physician or a consultant familiar with biochemical-based mental illness and who is committed to alternative and complementary approaches to health and healing. This individual should begin clinical biochemical testing to define the specific source of the problem. This individual should be familiar with the various forms of depression and which approaches are most effective for which forms of depression.

This professional should be knowledgeable of any side effects, drug-to-nutrient reactions, nutrient-to-nutrient interactions, and any age or gender issues that might influence treatment choices.

When choosing a physician or mental health professional, be sure to ask about his or her training and certifications. Just because a person is a medical doctor does not mean that he or she is skilled in dealing with mental or emotional issues, especially depression.

Avoid ideologues and practitioners with a rigid point of view on the causes and treatment of depression. We are all looking for a magic pill but more often than not the healing of depression is a process involving numerous factors. Sometimes an effective holistic program for one person might be a poor choice for another. In fact, an effective program for one person may even aggravate existing symptoms or cause other symptoms in another person.

If you decide to work under the guidance or care of an alternative health consultant or practitioner, check out the individual's training and professional background. There are many skilled practitioners who may not have traditional training. Many types of alternative therapies are learned in informal settings and may not require a license or certification. Self-diagnosis and self-treatment for biochemical-based depression should never be attempted.

It is seldom that one practitioner has the necessary skills to understand all of the variables involved in healing an individual's suffering from chronic depression. Choose or ask your family or friends to help you select a primary practitioner or coach who is willing to treat you as a partner in the process of healing your depression and is willing to work with other wellness and health professionals.

Week Three: Form Your Healing Team

The ideal approach to healing chronic depression is to create a team of practitioners who have a history of referring clients to other healthcare professionals, such as a herbalists, psychotherapists, meditation teachers, stress-management consultants, energetic healers, support groups, pastoral counselors, nutritional consultants, and nutritionally based psychiatrists for evaluation and monitoring of any medication. For example, research demonstrates that many individuals who suffer from chronic, biochemical-based clinical depression respond best to a treatment regime combining psychotherapy and medication. In these cases, it is important that the various practitioners are respectful of each other's talents and are open to discussing the client's progress and needs.

Of course, all therapies and therapists should be chosen with common sense and with caution.

Week Four: Obtain a Preliminary Evaluation and Diagnosis

Once your team has been organized, a primary evaluation should be conducted that includes a nutritional, medical, and psychiatric history; a blood and urine analysis that pays special attention to hormonal and/or nutritional information; and a physical exam. While this process is being conducted, you should be balancing your lifestyle in some of the basic ways addressed in Week One of the program.

Be consistent in adding positive lifestyle changes each day while eliminating destructive or negative patterns. If you are isolating yourself, come out of your shell and reach out to others for support. Do not give up hope.

Week Five: Obtain a Specialized Western Evaluation and Diagnosis

Depression is very treatable. If, by the end of the fourth week, there has not been an appreciable change in your emotional state, then it is advisable that your team explore some of the more complex factors that alone or in combination can cause depression. Effective healing of depression often requires a process of elimination as to what the key factor or factors are. The most common causative factors to be investigated include:

- High toxic metal levels, especially of mercury and lead.
- Glandular or hormone imbalances, especially low thyroid, estrogen-to-progesterone ratios, and low blood sugar.
- Obvious and subclinical nutritional deficiencies especially of magnesium, vitamin B$_6$, boron, chromium, glycine, and the essential fatty acids.

Diagnostic procedures to be explored should include:

- Vitamin, mineral, and essential fatty acid testing.
- Saliva testing to explore estrogen-to-progesterone ratios.
- Thyroid testing (T3 and T4 levels).
- Hypoglycemia testing (glucose tolerance test).
- Allergy testing.
- Candida testing.
- Personality evaluation.
- Postural analysis.

At this stage, you are like a detective searching for the culprit of the crime. Seek out the clues. Do not give up hope. Just go through this process step by step and you will see the light at the end of the tunnel.

Week Six: Obtain a Specialized Energetic-Vibrational Evaluation and Diagnosis

An energetic-vibrational evaluation includes tools popular in Chinese medicine, Ayurveda, and homeopathy. This type of evaluation can include pulse, chakra, facial, and tongue evaluation, as well as applied kinesiology muscle testing. A properly performed evaluation can help determine if an undiagnosed medical problem is related to the depression.

This is an evaluation process based on faith and curiosity. Energetic-vibrational evaluations connect to your inner creativity and the passion for living fully.

Week Seven: Start the Western Therapeutic Process

Once the diagnostic and evaluation process is done, the therapeutic team, the patient, and his or her family can decide the best approach to embark on. This may require an inpatient component and special outpatient services for the patient and his or her family. Specialized therapy programs may also be helpful especially if organized within a supportive, structured therapeutic environment that facilitates medical and psychiatric treatment of depression. The goal of treatment is to restore the individual to effective functioning in addition to helping him or her to attain a more satisfactory psychological and social adjustment.

Week Eight: Start the Energetic Therapeutic Process

Once the energetic diagnostic and evaluation process is done, the therapeutic team (which might include polarity therapists, Reiki masters, pastoral counselors, and other natural healing specialists), the patient, and the family can decide the best approach to embark on.

When applying this approach, it is helpful to also work with a Western team that is open to alternative approaches. Do not expect instant results. Do not give up hope, but rather, be an active part of your own healing process. Go through this process patiently and communicate your needs to both your Western and your energetic healing team.

Week Nine: Begin a Diet and Supplement Program

The Emotional Healing Program is based primarily on the combining of a wide range of approaches that will rebalance brain biochemistry, and allow and support corrective perceptual processing of information. In addition, the program will help you develop effective coping strategies to reduce depression, without stress or anxiety, as well as enhancing your sense of emotional balance and well-being.

A central aspect of this healing program consists of a regulated diet, and nutritional and herbal supplementation to build up brain chemicals, such as serotonin and norepinephrine, that affect mood and are often abnormal in depressed people. Body detoxification, exercise, energy balancing, aromatherapy, homeopathy (including the Flower Remedies), scientific relaxation, and meditation are all tools of great value in healing depression.

This program is not designed to be rigid. Since there are so many types and causes of depression, you will have to explore what is best for you. A good way to start is to integrate one or two of the following diet or supplement suggestions. Individual characteristics such as sex, age, family history, and metabolic condition all determine emotional health. You can certainly integrate this program into whatever treatment program you are following, including one that uses antidepressant medication. If you are on medication, discuss it with your physician or mental health professional.

Begin Taking Selected Nutritional and Herbal Supplements

Explore the supplements that have been discussed throughout the book. You might get relief from depression by replacing essential fatty acids to create PGE1, restoring key vitamins and minerals, treating hypothyroidism, correcting hypoglycemia, avoiding foods and chemicals responsible for cerebral allergy and sensitivity, or treating an existing candida-related problem.

The dosage and effectiveness of any therapeutic approach including drugs will be influenced by metabolism, weight, physical health, and the depth of the depression. Self-treatment can be dangerous and at times even fatal. Some nutrients, though safe in small amounts, can be toxic if taken in high doses. As discussed earlier, what may be a normal dosage for one person may be high for another.

Begin a Specialized Diet

Build your program around foods low on the glycemic index. If you are found to have candida or food sensitivities, adjust the foods you choose accordingly.

Eliminate those foods or chemically addictive substances that might be part of the cycle leading to your depression. If low blood sugar is the cause of your depression, create a dietary and supplementation program to balance your adrenal and pancreatic function.

Plan Your Carbohydrate Intake

Just as with protein, when you eat carbohydrates is critical to how your brain will respond. Timing is everything. Here is a basic meal plan to follow:

Breakfast

Begin the day with a mixture of protein and complex carbohydrates: low-fat milk or soymilk with whole-grain cereal and fresh fruit. You can even eat multi-whole-grain pancakes.

Lunch

To renew mental energy for the afternoon, have a salad with low-fat dressing made with soy mayonnaise or yogurt. Tofu, a vegeburger, or any combination of grains and beans is also filling and nutritious.

Afternoon Snack

Use the midday snack to supply your brain with carbohydrates. Choose a piece of fresh fruit or low-fat whole-grain crackers and vegetable juice cocktail.

Dinner

Start the evening with a complex carbohydrate such as a baked potato, squash, or corn as a side dish. Choose a choline-rich food such as lentil soup for your entrée, and finish you meal with a low-fat frozen yogurt dessert.

Bedtime Snack

Relax your brain and prepare for a good night's sleep with tryptophan-rich warm low-fat milk with a little tupelo honey and a banana.

Week Ten: Observe Your Daily Patterns

Are your more energetic in the morning, afternoon, or evening? Moods are known to generally be higher in periods when you have more energy and lower when you are less energized. Learn techniques to replenish your energy. When you are able to anticipate events or patterns that cause fatigue, you can avoid them or better prepare yourself for them nutritionally and psychologically.

Week Eleven: Begin an Emotional Healing Program

As your symptoms improve, it is important that you begin a consistent program of balanced emotional-spiritual counseling This can include meditation, attitudinal counseling, creative expression exercises, humor therapy, and stress-management counseling. Consider working with a cognitive-behavioral therapist, a family therapist, a pastoral counselor, or a Gestalt therapist. Also consider relationship counseling or entering Freudian or Jungian analysis. You can also explore childhood trauma by taking a workshop with John Bradshaw or someone who specializes in healing the "inner child."

As part of your program, you might wish to:

- Practice meditation-visualization techniques.
- Exercise daily.
- Find a quiet, secluded place when you are surrounded by noise, smoke, and crowds of people.
- Call a friend for a chat or have a conversation with a colleague or coworker when confronted with the stress of loneliness. You can discuss or develop an idea or create a solution for a problem you have been working on.
- Develop close, supportive personal relationships. If you do not know how to do this or are frightened by the idea of giving up your independence, consider discussing this as part of your professional counseling.
- Take three-minute minibreaks throughout your workday. If you can find a place to lie down and raise your feet above your head, this can be very relaxing.
- Listen to quiet, soothing music through a portable Walkman cassette player.
- Take a short walk.
- Take a fifteen-minute nap.
- Do deep breathing and relaxation exercises.
- Take classes on time management.
- Learn self-massage or acupressure.
- Join a support group or seek professional guidance from a stress-management consultant.
- Have a massage or acupressure session.

Week Twelve: Some Additional Healing Options

Healing is a path, a jigsaw puzzle, a map to unknown but wonderful places. It is a search engine to the soul, a friend, a motivator, food for the spiritually starving, air for the suffocating mind.

It is a path that is not easily mapped. Lines are constantly being drawn and redrawn. The territories defined by these lines are full of gray areas, comfort zones, and obvious conflicts—the distinction between emotional intuition and the intellectual obvious.

There is no strict definition of natural healing or alternative and complementary medicine. The systems and techniques that are often considered "natural" are not always reasonable, practical, sensible, or rational. However, these natural systems and techniques will nudge you to see yourself more clearly by correcting and heightening your understanding of the causes of and effective treatment approaches for depression.

Following are twelve things you can review or add to your program:

- Self-healing. Explore the Bach Flower Remedies, aromatherapy, color therapy, light therapy, and sound and music therapy. Begin a body purification program.
- EEG-biofeedback, meditation, visualization, hypnosis, and brain machine technology. Harness your mind to heal your mind. Use NAET to reduce allergies.
- Art therapy, music therapy, and movement and dance therapy. All of these can help you express your emotions more easily without words. Creative expression is a powerful path out of depression.
- Support groups. Twelve-step programs can be invaluable for freeing yourself from emotional and physical addictions.
- Exercise. Develop a consistent daily program. Try walking, weight lifting, bike riding, yoga, or tai chi.
- Improving your external environment. Take a class on feng shui, change the colors in your home, buy plants, or maybe even put in a small portable waterfall.
- Hands-on healing and bodywork, polarity therapy, massage, Reiki, cranial-sacral work, and deep emotional release techniques. These are all powerful healing tools for emotional imbalance and stress.

Generally speaking, if a person experiences depression that is the result of a biochemical imbalance, one of two things will take place in the course of applying an integrated program. Either the imbalance will be corrected and the individual will eventually reduce his or her dosages of nutrition factors, or the imbalance will be found to be due to some other factor. In the latter case, a consistent wellness program that will bring about a permanent healing from depression is recommended. In rare cases, a genetic factor may underlie the depression. In such a case, any effective program will have to be continued with some adjustments for a long time, even years, or for the rest of the person's life. Even in such a case, many benefits can be expected, including the reduction or elimination of the symptoms associated with depression.

12 ❧ Some Final Thoughts

The traditional medical approach to depression is to find the symptom, decide which drug will work best to get rid of the symptom, treat that symptom, and discharge the client/patient. In such an approach, antidepressant medications of various dosages in various combinations are prescribed as a matter of course with virtually no attention being paid to those factors that created the symptom to begin with. This happens for a number of reasons but more than anything else the fact remains that drugs are cheaper and less time-consuming than emotional and spiritual counseling, preventive medicine, or lifestyle adjustment on the part of the client/patient.

Antidepressant medications are much easier to promote both to the consumer and to the typical family doctor. Prescriptions take less time and effort than dialogue, evaluation, diagnosis, and inquiry. Prescribing a drug takes less time and effort than organizing a class on wellness or exploring the support systems and family dynamics that cause an individual to continue emotionally toxic or disease-producing lifestyle patterns.

Though there are certainly situations where extreme medical intervention (drugs and surgery) are necessary, we live in a culture where medications are more often than not prescribed for people who don't need them. These medications will always be the first choice of treatment simply because they are available, and the selling of immediate gratification is a key element in our culture. This culture as a way of life leads directly to personal irresponsibility. These issues combined with the tunnel vision of the orthodox medical establishment will always create a symptom-drug partnership that is unrelated to real healing and a proactive, productive healthcare culture.

Many physicians question the validity of alternative approaches to the treatment of depression. They often argue that the treatments have no rational or scientific basis and have not been clinically tested through traditional scientific methods. This criticism is inappropriate because, unlike vitamins, amino acids, and pharmaceuticals, many integrated approaches to depression are difficult to do clinical research on, or test in the traditional scientific manner. How does one design a study, or set up a comparison group of persons, in order to evaluate the combined effects of various herbs, meditation, dance therapy, vitamins, and isolated amino acids on depression and different associated symptoms experienced by individuals of very different personalities?

These same critics attack concepts such as balancing of *chi*, emotional release bodywork, and other techniques that may be based in folk medicine, or spiritual inquiry. The truth is that as valuable as structural chemistry and pharmacology are to the development of therapeutic drugs and even some nutritional and amino acid therapies, many effective healing tools are the result of folk knowledge based on empirical verification and careful observation over hundreds, even thousands, of years. Sadly, many doctors who favor a more holistic, balanced approach to treating depression are reluctant to do so out of fear. Though the political environment at this time is freer for the practice of complementary, integrative, and holistic medicine and healing, there are always reports popping up in the media of physicians being censured by their medical boards, and even losing their licenses to practice.

According to *Blues Buster*, any factor that influences the neurohormones that control the stress response, and enable the body to more effectively respond to the physical and psychological changes that come with stress, may also reduce many of the symptoms associated with depression.[1]

Thus, in spite of the resistance to ideas presented in this book, it is important that everything be done to help an individual to free him- or herself from the prison of depression without causing greater harm. Simply taking antidepressant medication as the first response or ignoring the emotional history or chemical factors that have brought this condition about is the worst type of intervention. If medication is necessary, it should always be offered as part of a larger process that addresses these other causative issues.

NOTES

Chapter 1

1. *Blues Buster* (*Psychology Today*'s newsletter about depression), December 2001–January 2002.
2. Daniel Goleman, "Depression in the Old Can Be Deadly, but the Symptoms Are Often Missed," *The New York Times*, 6 September 1995.
3. Personal interview.
4. Ibid.
5. Warren E. Leary, "Depression as an Underlying Cause of Other Medical Problems," *The New York Times*, 17 January 1996.
6. *Blues Buster* (*Psychology Today*'s newsletter about depression), December 2001–January 2002.
7. Ibid.
8. *Psychology Today*, November–December 2002.
9. Leary, op. cit.
10. *PTypes—Personality Types*, http://geocities.com/ptypes/.
11. ABCNews.com.

Chapter 2

1. Warren E. Leary, "Depression as an Underlying Cause of Other Medical Problems," *The New York Times*, 17 January 1996.
2. *Dr. Parcells Center of Energy Healing.com*, http://www.parcellscenter. com.
3. "Parasitic Diseases and Your Health," *NutriTeam*, http://www.nutriteam. com/parasites.htm.
4. Ibid.
5. Ibid.

Chapter 3

1. "Kava-Kava Extract XS 1490 Versus Placebo in Anxiety Disorders," *Pharmacopsychiatry*, vol. 30, no. 1 (January 1997), pp. 1–5.

2 *Journal of the American Medical Association*, 15 April 1998.

Chapter 4

1. J. R. Hibbeln and N. Salem, Jr., "Dietary Polyunsaturated Fatty Acids and Depression: When Cholesterol Does Not Satisfy," *American Journal of Clinical Nutrition*, vol. 62, no. 1 (July 1995), pp. 1–9.

2. Charles Bates, *Essential Fatty Acids and Immunity in Mental Health* (Laguna Hills, CA: American College of Advancement in Medicine Conference, 1987).

3. "Bottled Water: Pure Drink or Pure Hype?," *Natural Resources Defense Council*, http://www.nrdc.org/default.asp.

4. *Journal of the American Medical Association*, vol. 213, no. 2 (13 July 1970), pp. 272–75.

5. Carl C. Pfieffer, *Mental and Elemental Nutrients* (New Canaan, CT: Keats Publishing, 1976).

6. Ibid.

7. *Tufts University Health and Nutrition Newsletter*, vol. 15, no. 9 (November 1997).

8. *Journal of Neuropsychiatry and Clinical Neuroscience*, vol. 8, no. 2 (Spring 1996), pp. 168–71.

9. Ray Sahelian, *Pregnenolone: Nature's Feel Good Hormone* (Garden City Park, NY: Avery Publishing Group, 1997).

10. Personal interview.

Chapter 5

1. Harvey M. Ross, *Fighting Depression*, Second Edition (New York: Contemporary Books, 1992).

2. John Lee, *What Your Doctor May Not Tell You About Premenopause: Balance Your Hormones and Life from Thirty to Fifty* (New York: Warner, 1996).

3. O. Agid, A. Y. Shalev, and B. Lerer, *Journal of Clinical Psychiatry*, vol. 62, no. 3 (2001), pp. 169–73.

4. Im Jackson, *Thyroid*, vol. 8, no. 10 (October 1998), pp. 951–56.

5. D. McGuire and Lynanne McGuire, *Journal of Abnormal Psychology*, vol. 111 (2002), pp. 192–97.

Chapter 6

1. G. H. Dodd and S. Van Toller, *Perfumery: The Psychology and Biology of Fragrance* (Norwell, MA: Chapman and Hall, 1990), p. 169.
2. M. Stoddart, *The Scented Ape* (New York: Cambridge University Press, 1990), p. 135.
3. Natalie Angier, "Powerhouse of Senses: Smell, at Last Gets Its Due," *The New York Times*, 14 February 1995.

Chapter 8

1. Lewis Harrison, unpublished manuscript.
2. Nancy Rosanoff, *Intuition Workout: A Practical Guide to Discovering and Developing Your Inner Knowing* (Santa Rosa, CA: Aslan Publishing, 1991), pp. 17–18.
3. Margaret Talbot, "The Placebo Prescription," *The New York Times Magazine*, 9 January 2000.
4. *Nutrition*, vol. 17, no. 9 (2002): pp. 709–12.
5. "Work, Sex and Prayer in America: So Much Solemn Faith, So Little Religious Loyalty" in "Health and Behavior" column, *Life*, 16 February 1999.
6. Judith Hooper and Dick Teresi. *Would the Buddha Wear a Walkman? A Catalog of Revolutionary Tools for Higher Consciousness* (New York: Fireside, 1990).
7. Ibid.
8. Ibid.
9. "The Role of Prayer in Healing," *Alternative Complementary Therapies*, vol. 1, no. 6 (November–December 1995), p. 351.
10. Harrison, op. cit.
11. Joan Barysenko, *The Beginner's Guide to Meditation* (audiocassette), 1998.
12. *ABC Online*, http://www.abc.net.au, 16 April 2002.
13. Kurt Goldstein, *The Organism* (New York: Zone Books, 1995).
14. *Nicole Pascal Motivational Designs,* http://www.motivationaldesigns.com.

Chapter 9

1. *Callahan Techniques,* http://tftrx.com/callahan.htm.
2. Net Mind Body.com, http://netmindbody.com/index_ie.html.
3. *Doctor's Guide,* http://www.docguide.com/dgc.nsf.

Chapter 10

1.   Sarah Powers, "Answering the Call," *Yoga Journal Online,* http://www.yoga-journal.com/wisdom/650_1.cfm.
2.   James Ray, *Journey of Power,* http://www.jamesray.com.
3.   Ibid.
4.   Personal interview.
5.   Katsusuke Tsubo Serizawa, *Vital Points for Oriental Therapy* (Tokyo: Japan Publications, 1976).
6.   *Ayrmetes: Advanced Cognitive Technologies,* http://www.ayrmetes.com/Products/testimony.htm.
7.   *Blues Buster* (*Psychology Today's* newsletter about depression), December 2001–January 2002.
8.   Ibid.
9.   Fran J. Levy, Judith Pines Fried, and Fern Leventhal, Editors, *Dance and Other Expressive Art Therapies: When Words Are Not Enough* (New York: Routledge, 1995).
10. Personal interview.
11. Andrew Solomon, *The Noonday Demon: An Atlas of Depression* (New York: Scribner, 2002).

Chapter 12

1.   *Blues Buster* (*Psychology Today's* newsletter about depression), December 2001–January 2002.

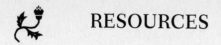 # RESOURCES

The following are the associations, books, journals, magazines, and websites that I consulted to preparing this book and that I recommend to anyone looking for additional information. Also included in the list are a number of treatment facilities for depression and depression-related disorders, and distributors to contact if you have problems obtaining some of the equipment used for the therapies discussed in this book.

Associations

Energetic and Vibrational Healing

American Polarity Therapy Association (APTA)
2888 Bluff Street
Suite 149
Boulder, CO 80301
Telephone: 303-545-2080

General

The National Institute of Mental Health
Information Resources and Inquiries Branch
5600 Fishers Lane
Room 7C-02
Rockville, MD 20857
Telephone: 301-443-4513

Humor Therapy

Gesundheit! Institute Hospital Foundation
P.O. Box 98072
Washington, DC 20090-8072
Website: www.patchadams.org

Association for Applied and Therapeutic Humor
1951 West Camelback Road
Suite 445
Phoenix, AZ 85015
Telephone: 602-995-1454
Fax: 602-995-1449
E-mail: office@aath.org

Pastoral Counseling

American Association of Pastoral Counselors (AAPC)
9504 Lee Highway
Fairfax, VA 22031
Telephone: 703-385-6967

Stress

Sedona Training Associates
60 Tortilla Drive
Sedona, AZ 86336
Telephone (information): 928-282-3522
Telephone (orders): 888-282-5656
Fax: 928-203-0602
E-mail: info@sedona.com

Thyroid

Broda O. Barnes, M.D., Research Foundation, Inc.
P.O. Box 110098
Trumbull, CT 06611
Telephone: 203-261-2101
Fax: 203-261-3017
E-mail: info@BrodaBarnes.org

Books and Articles

Aromatherapy

Angier, Natalie. "Powerhouse of Senses: Smell, at Last Gets Its Due." *The New York Times*, 14 February 1995.

Lawless, Julia. *Aromatherapy and the Mind*. London: Thorsons, 1995.

Lorig, T. S. "Cognitive and Non-Cognitive Effects of Odor Exposure: Electrophysical and Behavioral Evidence." In S. Van Toller and G. H. Dodd, Editors, *Fragrance: The Psychology and Biology of Perfume* (St. Louis, MO: Elsevier Science Publications, 1992).

Steele, J. "Brain Research and Essential Oils." *Aromatherapy Quarterly*, Spring 1984.

Worwood, Valerie Ann. *The Fragrant Mind*." Novato, CA: New World Library, 1996.

Bach Remedies

Bach, Edward. *Heal Thyself*. Saffron Walden, Essex, England: C. W. Daniel Company, 1931.

Bach, Edward. *The Twelve Healers and Other Remedies*. Saffron Walden, Essex, England: C. W. Daniel Company, 1936.

Weeks, Nora. *The Medical Discoveries of Edward Bach*. New Canaan, CT: Keats, 1973.

Bodywork, Massage, and Hands-On Healing

Harrison, Lewis. *Hands-On Healing*. New York: Kensington Books, 1998.

Pratt, George J., and Peter T. Lambrou. *Instant Emotional Healing: Acupressure for the Emotions*. New York: Broadway Books, 2000.

Candida

Crook, W. *There Are Better Ways to Help These Children*. Booklet. Jackson, TN: International Health Foundation, n.d.

Crook, William G. *The Yeast Connection: A Medical Breakthrough*. Jackson, TN: Professional Books, 1983, 1984, 1986.

Haas, A., et al. "The 'Yeast Connection' Meets Chronic Mucocutaneous Candidiasis." *New England Journal of Medicine*, vol. 314 (1986).

Truss, C. O. "The Role of Candida Albicans in Human Illness." *Journal of Orthomolecular Psychiatry*, vol. 10 (1981).

Chemical and Environmental Sensitivities

Barrett, S. "An Analysis of the National Environmental Justice Advisory Council Enforcement Subcommittee's Resolution #21 on Multiple Chemical Sensitivity." *Quackwatch*, www.Quackwatch.org., 20 August 2000.

Gots, R. E. *Multiple Chemical Sensitivities: What Is It?* North Bethesda, MD: Risk Communication International, 1993.

Staudenmayer, H. "Multiple Chemical Sensitivities or Idiopathic Environmental Intolerances: Psychophysiologic Foundation of Knowledge for a Psychogenic Explanation." *Journal of Allergy and Clinical Immunology*, vol. 99 (1997).

Chinese Medicine

Carter, Brian Benjamin. "Chinese Herbal Prozac: Depression and Traditional Chinese Medicine." *Acupuncture.com*, http://acupuncture.com, 2001.

Ren, Zhuoling. "Traditional Chinese Medicine and Depression," Part 2. *Edge News*, http://edgenews.com.

Cognitive-Behavioral Therapy

Beck, Aaron T., and A. John Rush. "Cognitive Therapy." In Harold I. Kaplan and Benjamin J. Sadock, Editors, *Kaplan and Sadock's Comprehensive Textbook of Psychiatry*, Fourth Edition, Volume 2 (Baltimore: Williams & Wilkins, 1985).

Detoxification

Harrison, Lewis. *30-Day Body Purification*. Upper Saddle River, NJ: Prentice-Hall Press, 1994.

Exercise, Movement, Yoga, and Dance

Brody, Jane. "Dancing Shoes Replace the Therapist's Couch." *The New York Times*, 18 October 1995.

Funderburk, James. *Science Studies Yoga: A Review of Physiological Data.* Honesdale, PA: Himilayan International Institute, 1977.

Levy, Fran J. *Dance Movement Therapy: A Healing Art.* Reston, VA: American Alliance for Health, Physical Education, Recreation and Dance, 1988.

General

Berfield, Susan. "A CEO and His Son: A Journey of Depression and Hope." *BusinessWeek*, 27 May 2002.

Blues Buster. Psychology Today's newsletter about depression. December 2001–January 2002.

Brody, Jane. "Dysthymia (Pronounced dis-THIGH-mee-a)." *The New York Times*, 18 January 1995.

Burns, David D. *The Feeling Good Handbook.* New York: Plume, 1999.

Cronkite, Kathy. "On the Edge of Darkness: Conversations About Conquering Depression." *Los Angeles Times/BusinessWeek.*

Gilbert, Paul. *Overcoming Depression: A Step-by-Step Approach to Gaining Control over Depression*, Second Edition. New York: Oxford University Press, 2001.

Goldstein, Kurt. *The Organism: A Holistic Approach to Biology.* Salt Lake City, UT: Zone Books, 1939.

Leary, Warren E. "Depression as an Underlying Cause of Other Medical Problems." *The New York Times*, 17 January 1996.

Norden, Michael J. *Beyond Prozac: Brain-Toxic Lifestyles, Natural Antidotes and New Generation Antidepressants.* New York: Regan Books, 1996.

O'Connor, Richard. *Undoing Depression: What Therapy Doesn't Teach You and Medication Can't Give You.* New York: Berkley Publishing Group, 1999.

Perry, Angela R., Editor. *American Medical Association Essential Guide to Depression.* New York: Pocket Books, 1998.

Roberts, Marjorie. "Depression: The Cry from Deep Within." *Let's Live Magazine*, August 1981.

Ross, Harvey M. *Fighting Depression*. New Canaan, CT: Keats Publishing, 1992.

Solomon, Andrew. *The Noonday Demon: An Atlas of Depression*. New York: Scribner, 2002.

Thayer, Robert E. *Calm Energy*. New York: Oxford University Press, 2001.

"When God Hides His Face." *Time*, 16 July 2001.

Herbs

Arora, D. S., and J. Kaur. "Anti-Microbial Activity of Spices." *International Journal of Antimicrobial Agents*, vol. 12 (1999).

Balick, Michael, and Paul Alan Cox. *People, Plants, and Culture: The Science of Ethnobotany*. Columbus, OH: W. H. Freeman and Company, 1997.

Hammer, K. A., C. F. Carson, and T. V. Riley. "In-Vitro Activity of Essential Oils, in Particular *Melaleuca Alternafolia* (Tea Tree) Oil and Tea Tree Oil Products, Against Candida Albicans." *Journal of Antimicrobial Chemotherapy*, vol. 42 (1998).

Harrison, Lewis. *Helping Yourself with Natural Healing*. Upper Saddle River, NJ: Prentice-Hall Publishers, 1989.

Tierra, Michael. "Standardized Herbal Extracts: An Herbalist's Perspective. *The New York Times Online*, www.nytimes.com, 1995.

Truss, C. Orian. *The Missing Diagnosis*. Birmingham, AL: Missing Diagnosis, 1983.

Light and Color Therapy

Graham, Helen. *Discover Color Therapy*. Berkeley, CA: Ulysses Press, 1998.

Ott, John. *Health and Light*. New York: Pocket Books, 1973.

Rosenthal, Norman. *Winter Blues: Seasonal Affective Disorder*. New York: Guilford Press. 1998.

Medications

Graedon, Joe. *The People's Pharmacy*. New York, Avon Books, 1976.

Martin, Eric W. *Hazards of Medicine: A Manual on Drug Interactions, Incompatibilities, Contraindications, and Adverse Effects*. Philadelphia: Lippincott, 1971.

Music, Sound, and Tuning Forks

Beaulieu, John, Minsun Kim, Elliott Salamon, and George B. Stefano. "Sound Therapy Induced Relaxation: Down Regulating Stress Processes and Pathologies." *Medical Science Monitor* (2002).

Benz, Danielle, Patrick Cadet, Kirk Mantione, and George B. Stefano. "Tonal Nitric Oxide and Health." *Medical Science Monitor* (2002).

Dahl, M., E. Rice, and D. Groesbeck. "Effects of Fiber Motion on the Acoustic Behavior of an Anistropic Flexible Fibrous Membrane." *Journal of the Acoustical Society of America*, vol. 87 (1990).

Lenhardt, M., R. Skellett, P. Wang, and A. Clarke. "Human Ultrasonic Speech Perception." *Science*, vol. 253 (1991).

Sales, Alan. *Tuning Forks for Healing Therapy*. Bristol, Avon, England: Positive Health Publications, 1994-2002.

Stefano, George, B., Michael Salzetcde, and Harold I. Magazine. "Cyclic Nitric Oxide Release by Human Granulocytes, and Invertebrate Ganglia and Immunocytes: Nano-Technological Enhancement of Amperometric Nitric Oxide Determination." *Medical Science Monitor* (2002).

Nutritional Therapy

Benjamin, J., et al. "Double-Blind, Placebo-Controlled, Crossover Trial of Inositol Treatment for Panic Disorder." *American Journal of Psychiatry*, vol. 152 (1995).

Birkmayer, W., et al. "L-Deprenyl Plus L-Phenylalanine in the Treatment of Depression." *Journal of Neural Transmission*, vol. 159 (1984).

Brody, Theodore M., Joseph Larner, and Kenneth P. Minneman, Editors. *Human Pharmacology*. St. Louis, MO: Mosby International, 1998.

Goleman, Daniel. "Depression in the Old Can Be Deadly, but the Symptoms Are Often Missed." *The New York Times*, 6 September 1995.

Harrison, Lewis. *The Complete Fats and Oils Book*. New York: Avery, 1996.

Kravitz, Howard M., et al. "Dietary Supplements of Phenylalanine and Other Amino Acid Precursors of Brain Neuroamines in the Treatment of Depressive Disorders." *Journal of the American Osteopathic Organization*, supplement, vol. 84 (September 1984).

Linder, Maria C., Editor. *Nutritional Biochemistry and Metabolism*, Second Edition. Maidenhead, Berkshire, England: Appleton and Lange, 1991.

Pfeiffer, Carl C. *Mental and Elemental Nutrients*. New Canaan, CT: Keats Publishing, 1975.

Sabelli, H. C. "Rapid Treatment of Depression with Selegiline-Phenylalanine Combination." Letter. *Journal of Clinical Psychiatry*, vol. 52 (March 1991).

Sahelian, Ray. *Mind Boosters: A Guide to Natural Supplements That Enhance Your Mind, Memory, and Mood*. New York: St. Martin's Press, 2000.

Sahelian, Ray. *Pregnenolone: Nature's Feel Good Hormone*. New York: Avery, 1997.

Schmidt, Michael A. *Smart Fats: How Dietary Fats and Oils Affect Mental, Physical and Emotional Intelligence*. Berkeley, CA: Frog, 1997.

Shamsuddin, A. M. *Journal of Nutrition*, vol. 124 (1995), supplement.

Personality and Depression

Coan, R. W. "Personality Types." In R. J. Corsini, Editor, *Encyclopedia of Psychology*, Second Edition, Volume 3 (New York: Wiley, 1994).

Gunderson, John G. "Personality Disorders: Introduction." In Task Force on Treatments of Psychiatric Disorders, American Psychiatric Association, *Treatments of Psychiatric Disorders*, Vol. 3 (Washington, DC: American Psychiatric Association, 1989).

Katharine A. Phillips, et al. "Is Depressive Personality Disorder a Distinct Disorder?" *American Journal of Psychiatry*, vol. 155 (1998), pp. 1044–48.

Schwartz, M. A., O. P. Wiggins, and M. A. Norko. "Prototypes, Ideal Types, and Personality Disorders: The Return to Classical Phenomenology." In W. John Livesley, Editor, *The DSM-IV Personality Disorders* (New York: Guilford Press, 1998).

Widiger, T. A., and L. M. Sankis. "Adult Psychopathology: Issues and Controversies." *Annual Review of Psychology*, vol. 51 (2000).

Placebo

"Is the Placebo Powerless? An Analysis of Clinical Trials Comparing Placebo with No Treatment." *The New England Journal of Medicine*, vol. 344, no. 21 (24 May 2001).

Talbot, Margaret. "The Placebo Prescription." *The New York Times Magazine*, 9 January 2000).

Positive and Negative Ions

Karnstedt, Jim, and Don Strachan. "Negative Ions: Vitamins of the Air?" *Ion and Light,* http://www.ionlight.com/air/airarticles/negionvitamine sofair.html.

Soyka, Fred. *The Ion Effect.* Macclesfield, Cheshire, England: Bookthrift Company, 1977.

Prayer

Dossey, Larry. *Healing Words: The Power of Prayer and the Practice of Medicine.* New York: HarperCollins, 1993.

Dossey, Larry. *Prayer Is Good Medicine: How to Reap the Healing Benefits of Prayer.* New York: Harper and Row, 1996.

Larson, Cynthia Sue. "Prayer Is Good Medicine." *Reality Shifters,* http://realityshifters.com, 5 October 2000.

Progesterone-Estrogen Ratio

Lee, John. *What Your Doctor May Not Tell You About Menopause: The Breakthrough Book on Natural Progesterone.* New York: Warner, 1996.

Lee, John. *What Your Doctor May Not Tell You About Premenopause: Balance Your Hormones and Life from Thirty to Fifty.* New York: Warner, 1999.

Martin, Raquel. *The Estrogen Alternative: Natural Hormone Therapy with Botanical Progesterone,* Third Edition. Rochester, VT: Inner Traditions, 2000.

Sellman, Sherill. *Hormone Heresy: What Women Must Know About Their Hormones,* Revised. Tulsa, OK: GetWell International, 2000.

Relationships and Depression

Oxford, Linda, and Daniel J. Wiener. *Action Therapy with Families and Groups.* Washington, DC: American Psychological Association, 2003.

Wiener, Daniel J. *Rehearsals for Growth.* New York: W. W. Norton and Company, 1994.

St. John's Wort

"Inhibition of MAO and COMT by Hypericum Extracts and Hypericin." *Journal of Geriatric Psychiatry and Neurology*, vol. 7, supplement (1994).

Staffeldt, B., et al. "Pharmacokinetics of Hypericin After Oral Intake of the Hypericum Perforatum Extract LI 160 in Healthy Volunteers." *Journal of Geriatric Psychiatry and Neurology*, vol. 7, supplement (1994).

Suzuki, O., et al. "Inhibition of Monoamone Oxidase by Hypericum." *Planta Medica*, vol. 3 (1984).

Shilajit

"Antioxidant Defense by Native and Processed Shilajit: A Comparative Study." *Indian Journal of Chemistry*, vol. 35B (February 1996).

Bhattacharya, Salil K., and Ananda P. Sen. "Effects of Shilajit on Biogenic Free Radicals." *Phytotherapy Research*, vol. 9 (1995).

"Chemistry of Shilajit, an Immunomodmodulatory Ayurvedic Rasayan." *Pure and Applied Chemistry*, vol. 62, no. 7 (1990).

Stress

Agid, O., A. Y. Shalev, and B. Lerer. "Triiodothyronine Augmentation of Selective Serotonin Reuptake Inhibitors in Posttraumatic Stress Disorder." *Journal of Clinical Psychiatry*, vol. 62, no. 3 (2001).

Technology and Brain-Mind Machines for Reducing Depression

Hooper, Judith, and Dick Teresi. *Would the Buddha Wear a Walkman? A Catalogue of Revolutionary Tools for Higher Consciousness.* New York: Fireside Publishing, 1990.

Thyroid

Arem, Ridha. *The Thyroid Solution: A Mind-Body Program for Beating Depression and Regaining Your Emotional and Physical Health.* New York: Ballantine Books, 2000.

Barnes, Broda O., and Lawrence Galton. *Hypothyroidism: The Unsuspected Illness.* New York: HarperCollins, 1976.

Heuer, H., M.K.H. Schafer, and K. Bauer. "Thyrotropin-Releasing Hormone (TRH): A Signal Peptide of the Central Nervous System." *Acta Medica Austriaca*, vol. 26, no. 4 (1999).

Joffe, R. T. "Refractory Depression: Treatment Strategies, With Particular Reference to the Thyroid Axis." *Journal of Psychiatry and Neuroscience*, vol. 22, no. 5 (November 1997).

Konig, F., C. von Hippel, T. Petersdorff, and W. Kaschka. "Antithyroid Antibodies in Depressive Diseases." *Acta Medica Austriaca*, vol. 26, no. 4 (1999).

Langer, Stephen E., and James F. Scheer. *Solved: The Riddle of Illness*, Third Edition. New York: Contemporary Books, 2000.

Lasser, R. A., and R. J. Baldessarini. "Thyroid Hormones in Depressive Disorders: A Reappraisal of Clinical Utility." *Harvard Review of Psychiatry*, vol. 4, no. 6 (March–April 1997).

Rack, S. K., and E. H. Makela. "Hypothyroidism and Depression: A Therapeutic Challenge." *Annals of Pharmacotherapy*, vol. 34, no. 10 (2000).

Rosenthal, M. Sara, and Robert Volpe. *The Thyroid Sourcebook: Everything You Need to Know*, Fourth Edition. New York: Contemporary Books, 2000.

Sullivan, P. F., D. A. Wilson, R. T. Mulder, and P. R. Joyce. "The Hypothalamic-Pituitary-Thyroid Axis in Major Depression." *Acta Psychiatrica Scandinavica*, vol. 95, no. 5 (May 1997).

Weissel, M. "Treatment of Psychiatric Diseases with Thyroid Hormones." *Acta Medica Austriaca*, vol. 26, no. 4 (1999).

Distributors

Flower Remedies

Nelson Bach USA Ltd.
100 Research Drive
Wilmington, MA 01887
Telephone: 800-319-9151
E-mail: info@nelsonbach.com
International distributor of Bach Flower Remedies.

Dr. Edward Bach Centre
Mount Vernon
Bakers Lane
Sotwell, Oxon OX10 0PZ
England
Telephone: 44 (0) 1491 834678
Fax: 44 (0) 1491 825022
Website: www.bachcentre.com
International distributor of Bach Flower Remedies.

Light and Color Therapy

Amjo Corp.
P.O. Box 8304
West Chester, OH 45069
Telephone: 513-942-2770 or 877-289-2656
Fax: 513-942-2771
E-mail: info@amjo.biz
Website: http://www.homephototherapy.com/contact.htm
UVA and UVB phototherapy supplies.

Music, Sound, and Tuning Forks

Dr. John Beaulieu, N.D., Ph.D.
BioSonic Sound Healing Enterprises
P.O. Box 487
High Falls, NY 12440
Telephone: 845-687-4767, extension 232, or 800-925-0159
Fax: 845-687-0205
Website: www.BioSonicEnterprises.com
For tuning forks, Tibetan quartz bowls, and other sound-based healing tools.

Treatment Facilities

Academy of Natural Healing
E-mail: chihealer@mindspring.com
For general information.

Hazelden
15245 Pleasant Valley Road
P.O. Box 11—CO 3
Center City, MN 55012-0011
Telephone: 800-257-7800
Treats substance abuse as the primary diagnosis. Depression is handled within the context of and secondary to a primary recovery-based treatment focus.

Huxley Institute for Biosocial Research
1209 California Road
Eastchester, NY 10709

Life Healing Center
P.O. Box 6758
Sante Fe, NM 87502
Telephone: 800-989-7406
E-mail: lhc@life-healing.com
Targets persons with depression as a primary diagnosis and secondary issues with eating disorders, abuse, and so on.

The Meadows
1655 North Tegner Street
Wickenburg, AZ 85390
Telephone: 800-632-3697
Treats substance abuse and codependency and also addresses depression when it is the primary diagnosis.

Vanderbilt Phototherapy Center
608 Medical Arts Building
1211 21st Avenue South
Nashville, TN 37212-1226
Telephone: 615-936-0858
Website: http://www.mc.vanderbilt.edu/health/centers/photo.html
A phototherapy outpatient facility.

Websites

General

AlternativeMentalHealth.com
http://alternativementalhealth.com
This is the world's largest website devoted exclusively to alternative mental health treatments. It includes a directory of over 300 physicians, nutritionists, experts, organizations, and facilities around the United States that offer or promote safe, alternative treatments for severe mental symptoms. Many of the physicians listed do in-depth examinations to find the physical causes behind mental problems.

CAM on PubMed
www.nlm.nih.gov/nccam/camonpubmed.html
Database of science-based information.

FDA Center for Food Safety and Nutrition
www.cfsan.fda.gov

Federal Trade Commission
www.ftc.gov/bcp/menu-health.htm

National Center for Complementary and Alternative Medicine
http://nccam.nih.gov

National Center for Complementary and Alternative Medicine Clearinghouse
http://nccam.nih.gov/health/clearinghouse/

National Institutes of Health Office of Dietary Supplements
http://ods.od.nih.gov

Quackwatch
www.quackwatch.org
Though this website is critical of virtually every therapeutic approach described in this book and could not be considered in any way a friend of alternative medicine or natural healing, its mission statement is clear and the information it presents is well organized. Its mission, in part, "is to combat

health-related frauds, myths, fads, and fallacies. Its primary focus is on quackery-related information that is difficult or impossible to get elsewhere." It questions or attacks virtually every alternative or unorthodox approach to healing, including most aspects of Chinese medicine, chiropractic, and so on, saying that such techniques are unproven or lack scientific validity. If the ideas in this book seem too "alternative" for your tastes, you may want to check them out on Quackwatch. Quackwatch's worldview concerning health-care is based on a very strictly defined "scientific approach."

Hypnosis

Hypnosis.com
www.hypnosis.com
Lyle Tautfest answers questions about hypnosis.

Rehearsals for Growth

Rehearsals for Growth
www.rehearsals.com/RfG

Relationship Counseling

Mars and Venus Counseling Center
www.debraburrell.com

Seasonal Affective Disorder

Dr. Koop.com
http://www.drkoop.com/adam/peds/top/002394.htm

National Organization for Seasonal Affective Disorder
www.nosad.org

Stress

The Dr. Gabe Mirkin Show
http://DrMirkin.com
Dr. Mirkin offers health reports.

Writer's Block and Depression

Talk with a Writer
www.talkwithawriter.com
Jerry Mundis offers advice.

INDEX